Intra-Abdominal Infections
Pathophysiology and Treatment

Dietmar H. Wittmann

Medical College of Wisconsin
Milwaukee, Wisconsin

Marcel Dekker, Inc.   New York • Basel • Hong Kong

Library of Congress Cataloging-in-Publication Data

Wittmann, D. H. (Dietmar H.)
    [Intraabdominelle Infektinonen. English.]
    Intra-abdominal infections : pathophysiology and treatment / D. H.
  Wittmann.
        p.   cm.
    Translation of: Intraabdominelle Infektinonen.
    Includes bibliographical references.
    Includes index.
    ISBN 0-8247-8497-9 (alk. paper)
    1. Abdomen—Infections—Handbooks, manuals, etc. I. Title.
    [DNLM: 1. Abdomen—physiopathology. 2. Bacterial Infections—
physiopathology. 3. Bacterial Infections—therapy. 4. Digestive
System Diseases—physiopathology. 5. Digestive System Disease—
therapy. WI 900 W8321]
    RC944.W5513   1991
    617.5'5—dc20
    DNLM/DLC
    for Library of Congress

This book is printed on acid-free paper.

MARCEL DEKKER, INC.
270 Madison Avenue, New York, New York 10016

Current printing (last digit):
10 9 8 7 6 5 4 3 2 1

PRINTED IN THE UNITED STATES OF AMERICA

Didactic design:
Institut Mensch und Arbeit
Robert Pfützner GmbH, Munich, West Germany

Layout:
Prof. Fritz Lüdtke, Manuela Baur, Roland Beuck, Munich, West Germany

Introduction

Because intra-abdominal infections are still associated with a high patient morbidity and mortality, they remain a great surgical challenge. In this monograph Dr. Dietmar Wittmann has offered a complete, very well-organized review of the subject, including chapters on the clinical etiology of both peritonitis and intra-abdominal abscess, experimental studies that outline the probable pathophysiological events that occur in human disease, and the microbiology of intra-abdominal infections, including both the acute phase of peritonitis and the chronic phase of abscess.

An unusual feature of this book is a detailed approach to many of the scoring systems used to grade the severity of disease, including the Mannheim Peritonitis Index, the PIA II, and the APACHE II. The therapy section outlines the alternatives currently available in operative technique, choice of antibiotics, and other intensive-care decisions. The references are those most representative of the subject from both the United States and European literature. The abundant illustrations, graphs, and photographs help to keep the reader's interest level high and to emphasize the critical features of the subject.

Dr. Wittmann's book should be considered essential reading for practitioners who deal with intra-abdominal infections as well as for students who are studying microbiology, critical care, or surgery.

Ronald Lee Nichols, M.D., M.S.
Henderson Professor and Vice-Chairman
Department of Surgery
Tulane University School of Medicine
New Orleans, Louisiana

Presentation

The design of this book is intended to minimize reading time and increase the book's effectiveness for the reader. It departs from traditional scientific presentations in medicine, which are usually very complex. Normally, the reader has to work through the whole text before he can concentrate on the essentials. The goal here has been to highlight the essentials without sacrificing substance.

All passages in the text are weighted according to the following criteria:

In large type	Practice-oriented overview, evaluation, and significance of the following passages.
In medium type	Procedures with which the physician must be familiar.
In small type	Scientific commentary for selective reading.
Captions, tables, and graphs	Functional summaries and concise guides to decision making.
Digressions	Presentation of related fundamental topics for in-depth reading.
Bibliography	Additional literature is listed on pp. 76–81.
Reading time	Maximum 40 minutes for the main text in large and medium types. Time for additional texts depends on individual requirements.

Acknowledgments

Emphatic thanks are due to Dr. L. Frommelt of the Bacteriological Department of the General Hospital Hamburg-Altona and Dr. R. Fock of the Institute for Medical Microbiology and Immunology of the University of Hamburg for their assistance in preparing the bacteriological chapters and for the photography of bacteria.

I am especially grateful to Dr. E. Renatus of the Institut Mensch und Arbeit for her help in preparing and editing the German manuscript. Special thanks also go to Mrs. A. Sonntag of the General Hospital Hamburg-Altona for her outstanding photographic work. Additionally, I owe sincere thanks to Bonnie Jeanne Bates, Dr. Jack M. Bergstein, and Dr. Bernd G. E. Merkel, who helped me in preparing the English manuscript.

D. H. Wittmann

Contents

Intra-Abdominal Infections

Intra-abdominal infections are still an extremely difficult problem in surgery. Even today, the therapeutic challenge of intra-abdominal infections lies in their relatively high incidence and mortality rate.

Operative therapy can only partially eliminate the pathogens. Bacteria that have infected vital tissue must be removed by additional systemic antibiotic therapy. Intensive-care therapy will support the defensive mechanisms by controlling secondary damage to the organism.

In clinical practice, primary hematogenous, mainly monobacterial peritonitis is relatively rare compared to polymicrobial aerobic/anaerobic mixed infections due to intestinal perforation. Depending on the immune status of the organism, the infection will either remain localized as an abscess or diffuse into the whole peritoneal cavity.

Damage of intra-abdominal viscera precurses perforation and the massive influx of bacterial inocula into the peritoneal cavity. The localization and duration of this process determine the intensity of the defense reaction and of the entire infection. The infection is aggravated by an explosive increase of bacterial challenge. The often unfavorable local conditions and the synergistic pathogenicity of individual bacterial species, as well as prior damage to the total organism (comorbidity), rapidly lead to a breakdown of local defense mechanisms. The organism is taxed by pathogenetically significant injury, due to bacteria and their toxic metabolites, and by the body's own overreaction to inflammation. All organ systems are implicated and ultimately irreversibly damaged by the rapidly progressing and often uncontrolled reactions of the defense mechanism.

Therapeutic Strategy

1. **Elimination of the cause of infection**
2. **Removal of infective materials, necroses, and toxins**
3. **Optimization of defense mechanisms against infection**
4. **Treatment of the consequences of infection**

Surgery plays a key role in the treatment of peritonitis. Its objective is the elimination of the source of infection, thereby ending the influx of infective toxic material into the peritoneal cavity.

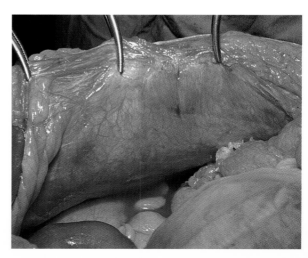

Inflammatory reaction of the peritoneum with edema and peritoneal exudate as well as hypervascularization of the peritoneum as an expression of acute inflammation.

Intra-abdominal infection is a bacterial inflammation that affects the visceral as well as the parietal peritoneum and may diffuse to neighboring tissues. The infection may disrupt the functioning of the entire organ system.

The terms *peritonitis* and *peritoneal inflammation* also encompass inflammations of the peritoneal cavity that are not primarily of bacterial origin. Strictly speaking, both terms refer only to a part of the total inflammatory reaction, which eventually involves the entire organism. In clinical practice, there is no clear differentiation between the terms *peritonitis* and *intra-abdominal infection*. The disease may progress from primarily nonbacterial inflammation to bacterial infections. It also includes intra-abdominal abscesses. In the following discussion, the terms *peritonitis* and *intra-abdominal infection* (IAI) will be used synonymously to indicate the spectrum of the disease.

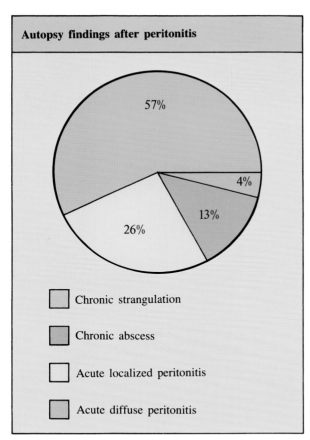

Autopsy findings after peritonitis

57%

4%

13%

26%

☐ Chronic strangulation

☐ Chronic abscess

☐ Acute localized peritonitis

☐ Acute diffuse peritonitis

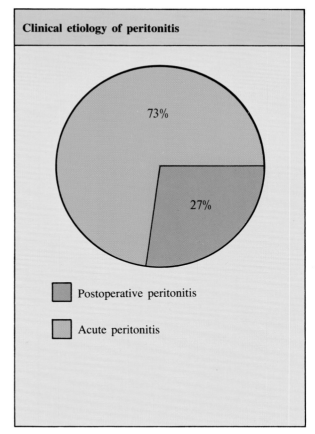

Clinical etiology of peritonitis

73%

27%

☐ Postoperative peritonitis

☐ Acute peritonitis

Incidence and Mortality of IAI

In representative autopsy findings at a German hospital, inflammation of the peritoneal cavity was noted in 897 of 11,000 patients; that is, 8%. In 56% of the cases, peritonitis was the sole cause of mortality; in 37% it was a major cofactor of death. As secondary findings intra-abdominal infections were of minor importance in only 6.3% of all cases.

Causes of Peritonitis

Most commonly, intra-abdominal infections are secondary to perforation of a hollow viscous organ. In 567 consecutive patients operated on for peritonitis at the General Hospital Hamburg-Altona, spontaneous perforation accounted for 73% of the cases, and postoperative perforation was seen in the remaining 27%.

Chronology of Treatment Results

The graph below documents the influence of individual therapeutic measures on mortality rates based on the weighted total mortality in the literature. The graph reflects the relative contributions of surgery, antibiotic therapy, and intensive care to the success of therapy.

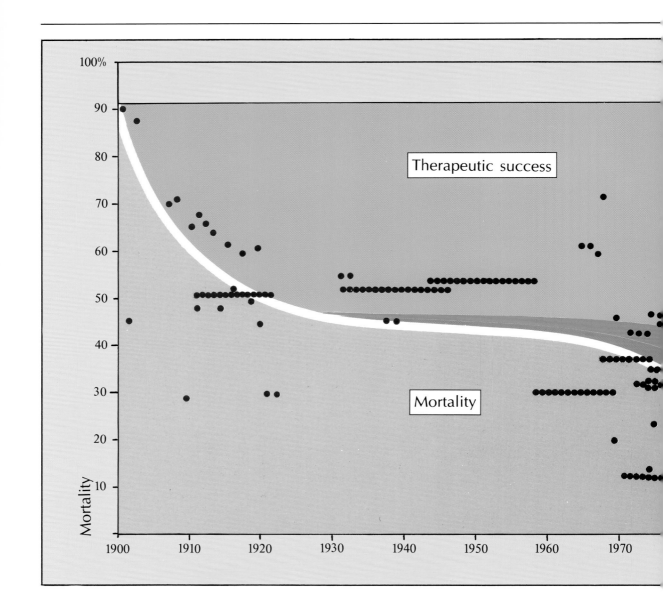

Incidence of Intra-Abdominal Infections

Over the past 50 years there has been a shift from peritonitis due to appendicitis to peritonitis originating from the large bowel. In comparison to earlier statistics, the incidence of intra-abdominal infections has changed insignificantly.

However, postoperative infections are seen more frequently. This, of course, is due to an increase in abdominal operations in patients of advanced age and with more risk factors. Moreover, new technical possibilities in surgery have pro-

moted this development. In part, the extension of indication also explains the meager progress in the management of peritonitis over the past 60 years.

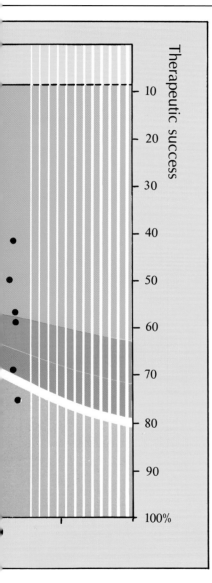

— 10
— 20
— 30
— 40
— 50
— 60
— 70
— 80
— 90
— 100%

Mortality reported over decades and fraction of therapeutic success attributable to operative management (green), antimicrobial therapy (red), and critical care management (blue).

Mortality

The mortality data are weighted according to the number of cases of peritonitis analyzed in publications by the following authors, from 1901 to 1980: Sudek, Körte, Kirschner, Braun, Kunz, Wachsmuth, Gall, Dinstl, Kiene, Eckert, Anders, Kern, Trede, Esser, Pheils, Weissenhofer, Herfarth, Altunbay, Goertz, Polk, Linder, Kern, Wittman, Häring, and others. (Each point on the graph represents 50 cases.)

Surgery

Thanks to systematization and strict administration of the principles Kirschner defined for the operative management of peritonitis at the 50th Annual Meeting of the Germany Society of Surgery in 1926, the mortality rate has dropped from 90% to below 50%. The literature for the subsequent four decades does not reveal any significant surgical–technical improvements.

Antibiotics

After the discovery of penicillin by Fleming and the subsequent development of broad-spectrum antibiotics, there was no significant therapeutic improvement. The available antibiotics were largely without effect on the pathogens causing peritonitis. Advances were finally made with the introduction of cephalosporins, totally inhibiting growth of the major endotoxin-producing bacteria, especially *E. coli*—and with the availability of antianaerobic compounds such as metronidazole and clindamycin.

Intensive-Care Therapy

Intensive-care therapy, which has become increasingly effective over the years, has gradually contributed to an improvement of survival rates for patients with intra-abdominal infections.

Recent Progress in Therapy

The following factors may be responsible for an improvement of therapy results:

The development of highly potent antibiotics effective against gram-negative bacteria, in particular *Escherichia coli* and *Bacteroides fragilis* as the relevant pathogens of intra-abdominal infections, and active in sufficiently high concentrations at the site of infection.

The general administration of efficient intensive-care therapy, which has led to an expansion of operative management, in turn reducing pathophysiological damage due to sepsis.

The optimization of surgical therapy for infections of the peritoneal cavity by adopting general principles for treating surgical infections (ubi pus, ibi evacua). Here, etappenlavage treatment has established itself as an elegant method. In this method the peritoneum is treated in stages and only temporarily closed, as a single operation cannot remove all foci. Thus, the infectious toxic material is eliminated in a stepwise procedure of scheduled reoperations, ultimately leading to complete control of the source of infection.

Chronology of Treatment Results

Optimized critical care and new antibiotics have led to decisive therapeutic advances in the past years. Nevertheless, the improved therapeutic situation cannot be regarded as satisfactory with regard to the results in treating intra-abdominal infections (IAI). Therefore, the

At the turn of the century, the mortality rate for peritonitis was between 80 and 90%. In 1926 Kirschner reported on the therapeutic results in Germany. He showed that the mortality rate could be continuously reduced by the strict implementation of surgical principles for treatment.

Therapeutic Milestones

Mortality

In 17 major studies since 1974, the mortality rates for all forms of peritonitis ranged from 13 to 43%. In evaluating these figures, one must bear in mind that individual authors have focused on different forms of peritonitis in different degrees of severity (for example, upper abdominal peritonitis following perforation of the biliary tract or gastroduodenal ulcers, peritonitis following perforated appendicitis, colon perforation or peritonitis following anastomotic dehiscence). Until recently, there was no uniform index allowing for direct comparison of the treatment of peritonitis. Each study based its mortality rates on different criteria, according to origin and pathogenesis of peritonitis. The recently established criteria are in the form of an index that allows a comparison between different treatment results. Nevertheless, the published figures in older studies still reveal a prognostic trend for this infectious disease. In this respect, the different definitions of peritonitis can be neglected, as they are about evenly distributed throughout all the studies.

Surgery

The systematic implementation of general surgical techniques and principles has reduced the mortality rate for peritonitis from 90 to 50%. The two major principles are:
- Elimination of the source of infection
- Removal of pus and infectious toxic material

When these measures were adopted, the mortality rate remained constant at first. Only after the introduction of more effective critical care and antibiotic therapy did a more aggressive surgical approach become possible, in particular, the open treatment as performed in the scheduled lavage (see pp. 58–63). As a result, the causes of peritonitis were addressed more efficiently, toxic material was removed, and pathophysiological changes leading to disease were controlled.

Nevertheless, the improved therapeutic situation cannot be regarded as satisfactory with regard to the results in treating IAI. Therefore, the search for improved methods in critical care and antibiotic therapy accompanying surgical procedures is mandatory.

search for improved methods in critical care and antibiotic therapy accompanying surgical procedures is mandatory.

The impact of antibacterial chemotherapy and intensive care was already addressed in Kirschner's report. However, in terms of mortality, therapeutic progress appears to have stagnated during the subsequent decades. Only since the mid 1970s have we been able to register further overall improvement in treatment results.

Antibiotics

After the discovery of penicillin by Fleming and the introduction of new broad-spectrum antibiotics in the therapy of peritoneal infections, there was no immediate improvement in treatment results. The mortality rates reported from the 1930s to the 1960s showed no improvement over the figures by Kirschner. In today's perspective, false hopes for the effectiveness of penicillins may have led to a neglect of surgical principles. This explains the high mortality rate during the postwar period. Not until the introduction of broad-spectrum penicillins and cephalosporins as well as substances active against anaerobic bacteria was there an improvement of treatment results clearly due to antibiotic therapy.

Critical Care

A number of factors have led to the improvement of critical-care therapy and thereby lowered mortality rates for IAI. These factors include: a better understanding of pathophysiological processes in damaged tissues and organs accompanying and following severe infections, the improvement of cardiopulmonary monitoring, computer-assisted analysis of circulatory parameters, and, finally, the rational use of old and new drugs. On the surgical side, these intensive measures have led to a more aggressive approach and contributed to the optimization of surgical treatment of peritoneal infections.

Therapeutic Strategies

In intra-abdominal infections all therapeutic measures have a common goal. Pathogenetically significant noxae are to be eliminated, and the damage caused by bacteria and the exotoxins and endotoxins of bacterial decomposition must be repaired. Recent debates on the optimal surgical-technical procedure in treating this disease must be seen in connection with the advances in critical care. These advances have undoubtedly expanded the possibilities of surgical therapy.

The accepted concepts for antimicrobial chemotherapy directed against causative agents remain problematic. We have yet to develop techniques that will inform the surgeon as to all the specific pathogens actually encountered. This information, however, is a prerequisite for optimal chemotherapy immediately after establishing diagnosis following incision for laparotomy. The discovery of penicillin in 1929 encouraged systemic and local application of antibiotics against intra-abdominal infections. Nevertheless—as measured by mortality curves—there was no immediate improvement of the prognosis for intra-abdominal infections upon routine application of antibiotics.

The Problem of Isolating Bacterial Agents

The identification of all causative agents requires special techniques, in particular since obligate anaerobes die off after only a brief exposure to air during their intraoperational isolation and subsequent procedures. Under routine clinical conditions, the methods necessary for isolation and identification of all etiologically relevant peritonitis pathogens are hardly feasible. Infectious material from the peritoneal cavity can seldom be applied to specific and selective nutrient media under oxygen-free conditions. Since all transport media are selective for specific bacteria, mainly *E. coli* and enterococci, they are unsuitable. Hence, bacteriological findings reported in the surgical literature over the past 40 years must be interpreted carefully. Although surgeons emphasized the importance of obligate anaerobes for the development of intra-abdominal infections at the beginning of the century, aerobic bacteria continued to be identified as the primary causative agents.

Perforation of the appendix is a typical source of intra-abdominal infection—22% of all peritonitis cases originate in the appendix. The infection can be life-threatening. Even today, the mortality rate is 13%.

A Typical Case History

At high seas on a Sunday evening, a 54-year-old ship's engineer suddenly experienced pain in the upper abdominal region. This was combined with nausea, later followed by vomiting. On Monday, the pain extended to the right lower abdomen. The patient developed low fever (38°C) and lost all appetite; vomiting did not recur. On Tuesday, he experienced severe pain in the entire abdomen, and his temperature rose to 39°C. On Thursday morning the patient was transferred to the nearest hospital.

Clinical Findings

Pulse rate over 120/min, blood pressure 100/60 mm Hg, respiration flat, with a respiration rate of 28/min.

The whole abdominal area was sensitive to pressure; rebound tenderness could be elicited in all four quadrants of the abdominal wall. Auscultation did not reveal bowel sounds.

Temperature 40.2°C; 18,400 leukocytes with shift to the left. Metabolic acidosis, increased serum urea level, serum creatinine 1.8 mg/dl, hypovolemia.

Surgery

The immediate laparotomy via transverse incision on the lower abdomen wall yielded 350 ml of pus from the entire abdominal cavity. The peritoneum was edematous and hypervascularized. A gangrenous appendix had led to intestinal perforation. Bacteria that had already become virulent during appendicitis had in-filtrated the peritoneal cavity. In addition, there was a thrombosis of the arteria appendicularis. Pus and tissue were immediately plated out on different culture media and placed in a gaspack system at 37°C for anaerobic cultivation. Gram staining revealed a mixed culture of gram-negative rods and gram-positive rods and cocci.

Immediately after diagnosis and removal of pus samples for bacteriological investigation, the anesthetist injected 2 g cefotaxime and 500 mg metronidazole.

The necrotic appendix was removed, its base ligatured and buried in the cecum. The peritoneal cavity was then washed with 10 L of Ringer's lactate until the drainage fluid ran clear. A spot drainage was positioned on the right lower side of the abdomen, and the peritoneal cavity was closed layer by layer.

Progress

On the first postoperative day, the patient's temperature dropped to 38°C, and it reached 37°C on the second postoperative day. The patient was artificially respirated and received a peridural catheter to avoid pain. Drainage yielded about 100 ml of clear peritoneal exudate daily. On the third postoperative day, breathing continued spontaneously and bowel activity resumed; on the fifth postoperative day, antibiotic therapy was discontinued. The patient resumed normal food intake. After primary healing of the wound and removal of stitches on the tenth postoperative day, the patient was well.

Clinical Symptoms and Their Determinants

Appendicitis presents typically: First, there is vague pain in the upper abdomen, accompanied by nausea. The pain then moves to the right lower abdomen. Finally, diffuse abdominal pain with rebound tenderness may occur.

The pathogenic sequence leads from local tissue damage to the in-

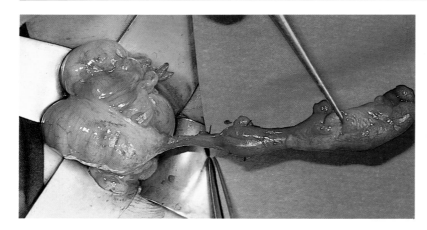

Acute appendicitis

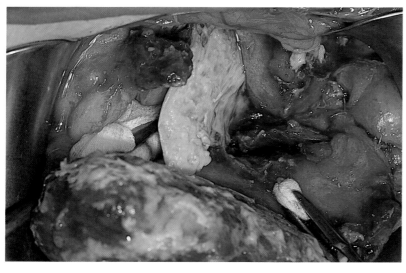

Appendix with tissue destruction, necrosis, and perforation.

What Has Happened Pathogenetically?

The necrosis of the appendix is promoted by septic thrombosis of the arteria appendicularis. In its anatomical function as functional end artery, this leads to a complete obstruction of the blood flow to the appendix. The necrotic and thus anaerobic tissue presents an ideal nutrient for obligate anaerobic bacteria and for a number of facultative anaerobes. The most commonly encountered pathogens are: *E. coli, Bacteroides fragilis, Clostridium perfringens,* peptostreptococci, and *Enterococcus faecalis.* The first sign of infection is the inflammatory reaction of the peritoneum surrounding the appendix due to the release of exotoxins by the pathogens. The visceral pain mediated by the autonomous nerve system is projected over the solar plexus and subsequently induces additional nausea and vomiting.

flammatory reaction of the periappendiculary peritoneum. Due to the decomposition of tissue by the activity of toxins combined with local acidosis and a breakdown in the supply of oxygen and nutrients, the local host defense mechanisms are kept at bay. As a result, diffuse peritonitis and septic shock occur.

Initially, local inflammatory reactions are heightened by the release of collagenases, hyaluronidases, and lecithinases, as well as other proteolytic and necrotizing enzymes. This is followed by local tissue necrosis in the inflamed area, in turn promoting the acidotic environment through a change in redox potential. Stimulated in their growth to release further toxins, the anaerobic bacteria favor a thrombosis of the arteria appendicularis. Finally, this results in a complete breakdown of oxygen and nutrient supply to the appendix. Such an occlusion also reduces or prevents the migration of the bloodborne host defenses to the site of infection.

The multiplication of bacteria, which to a certain degree act synergistically, proceeds uncontrolled. The flourishing bacteria are insufficiently held in check by the peritoneal defense system (omentum majus and fibrin formation = encapsulation of the abscess). Next, bacteria enter the peritoneal cavity (= diffuse peritonitis) and reach the central circulation via diaphragmatic lymphatic valves and thoratic lymphatic ducts. The consequences are bacteremia and endotoxinemia. When the patient described on p. 13 was admitted, these events were the basis of the clinical symptoms of septic shock.

The following table lists the typical bacteriological spectrum of intra-abdominal infections due to perforated appendicitis.

Bacteriology of Intra-Abdominal Infections Originating in the Appendix

Number of patients examined	$n = 61$
Bacteriological findings	n
E. coli	46
Klebsiella spp.	4
Proteus spp.	2
Citrobacter	1
Enterococcus faecalis	10
Streptococcus spp.	13
Staphylococcus aureus	1
Pseudomonas aeruginosa	7
Pseudomonas spp.	2
Other aerobes	6
Total	**92**
Candida	4
Bacteroides fragilis	36
Other Bacteroides	36
Fusobacterium spp.	2
Peptococcus spp.	6
Peptostreptococcus spp.	9
Clostridium perfringens	9
Clostridium spp.	2
Veillonella spp.	2
Other anaerobes	2
Total	**121**
Total number of isolated bacteria (including yeasts)	**217**

Source: Working Group on Peritonitis, Paul-Ehrlich-Society (1984).

3

Digression: What Is an Abscess?

The anatomical structure of abscesses with a firm fibrinous membrane due to lack of oxygen and nutrient supply implies anaerobic acidotic conditions in the abscess—ideal conditions for anaerobic growth.

An abscess is an accumulation of pus in an area where tissue has been destroyed. In the abdominal cavity, an abscess is separated from the healthy regions by fibrin capsule formation. Typically, an abscess characterizes the late stage of peritonitis in the presence of sufficient host defenses. The damaged tissue is melted away by bacterial and host enzymes. Suspended in the pus is necrotic tissue that has not been completely dissolved by phagocytes.

The severely reduced oxygen supply to the abscess implies pronounced anaerobic conditions and a low pH of 5.5 to 6.8. Ideal growth conditions for anaerobic bacteria in connection with increased osmolality lead to an influx of additional fluids into the abscess cavity, thereby increasing pressure. In this situation a spontaneous rupture of the abscess cavity can initiate a diffuse peritonitis. The concentrations of electrolytes, enzymes, and proteins in abscesses are shown in the table below.

Bacteriological investigations reveal up to twelve anaerobic bacteria types in the abscess cavity, for example, *Bacteroides fragilis, Fusobacterium necroforum, Bacteroides melaninogenicus, Peptococcus necrotisans, Clostridium perfringens,* and Clostridium species.

Although an abscess is often surrounded by a thick membrane, antibiotics can penetrate it. However, the effect of the substances in the acidic environment in the abscess cavity—particularly aminoglycosides—is greatly reduced. Other antimicrobials are inactivated in the abscess environment.

Physiology of Abscess Contents

	Mean value	Range	Unit
pH	6.2	5.5–6.8	
Osmolality	402	207–535	$\dfrac{mOsm}{kg\ H_2O}$
Glucose	86	0–233	mg/dl
Sodium	119	92–134	mg/dl
Potassium	18.5	10–33.5	mg/dl
Chloride	87.9	60–109	mg/dl
LDH	1417	51–3828	U/L
Total protein	4.5	1.3–7.5	g/dl
Albumin	1.7	0.6–6.0	g/dl

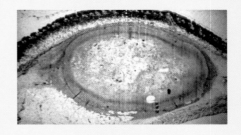

Microscopic section of a subcutaneous abscess: The abscess membrane ("capsule") is distinctly delineated. (Courtesy of Dr. John Bartlett, Johns Hopkins University School of Medicine.)

Pathophysiological Processes During Abscess Formation

Permeability increased

Pyogenic membrane

Exudation of protein

Fibrin formation

Tissue damage

Influx of phagocytes and macrophages

Bacterial growth

Death of phagocytes after 3-5 days

Release of Toxins and Enzymes

- Lipases
- Proteases
- Hyaluronidases
- Ribonucleases
- Leukosidines
- Hemolysins

Release of lysosomal enzymes + viable bacteria translocation

ABSCESS LIQUIFICATION

↑Osmolality
↓
↑**PRESSURE**

Accumulation of acidic metabolites
Substrate deficiency

O_2↓   PH↓ CO_2↑
ANAEROBIC ENVIRONMENT

Edema

Exterior to pyogenic capsule

| Vessels | Granulocytes | Mast cells | Fibrocytes |

These oxygen-consuming events support anaerobic conditions in the abscess and promote growth of obligate anaerobic pathogens, especially in light of diminished oxygen supply through the abscess membrane.

17

What Causes Necroses?

Necroses are caused by a diminished oxygen and nutrient supply in the course of mechanical and toxic damage to the tissue and nutrient-supplying vessels. Uncontrolled host defenses contribute to additional tissue damage.

Primary damage to living cells leads to necroses via mechanical damage or circulatory disturbances such as neoplastic tissue decomposition. The subsequent reduction of local defense mechanisms promotes the growth of bacteria found in the intestines that are normally controlled by host defense. These pathogens produce exotoxins (see table) in already damaged tissue.

The variety of tissue-damaging mechanisms reveals a complex pathophysiological picture in light of the myriad of pathogens. Research is only beginning to illuminate the interactions between individual bacteria species. Thanks to the interactions between bacterial metabolites, these pathogens escape from host defense mechanisms, reduce physiolog-

ical chemotaxis of neutrophils, and neutralize or destroy cellular defense. All these factors complicate research into the underlying mechanisms leading to necrosis and pus formation in the abscess.

Necrosis

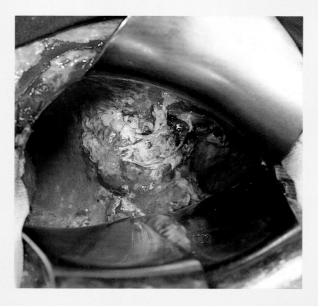

Examples of Exotoxins	
Exotoxin	**Pathogen**
Hemolysins	Peptostreptococci
Streptolysins	Aerobic and anaerobic Streptococci
Leukocidins	*Fusobacterium necroforum*
Cytoplasmatic toxins	*F. necroforum, Bacteroides fragilis,* Clostridiae
Cell wall–bound proteolytic enzymes	*B. fragilis*
Collagenases	Clostridiae, *B. melaninogenicus*
Hyaluronidases	Clostridiae
Heparinases	Enterobacteria, Fusobacteria, *B. fragilis*
Streptokinases and streptodornases	Aerobic and anaerobic Streptococci
Coagulases	Staphylococci, Streptococci, Clostridiae
Lecithinases	Clostridiae

Pus is mostly a mixture of leukocytes, dissolved tissue, and host as well as bacterial enzymes from which highly vital bacteria can be isolated.

In its pure form, pus consists of leukocytes that have migrated and will eventually die off due to steatosis. First minute fatty droplets, then larger ones, enter the protoplasm, while the nucleus breaks down into individual chromatin fragments. The fatty content of these particles lends pus the consistency and color (creamy and yellow to yellowish-green) of emulsified fats.

Large quantities of serous fluid lend pus a thin consistency described as seropurulent. Should pus be mixed with fibrin, it is referred to as fibrinous exudate. The presence of *Pseudomonas aeruginosa* is responsible for the greenish or bluish color of pus. Streptococci form a watery grayish pus, whereas a pure staphylococcal pus is thicker and creamy-yellow.

Blood lends pus its reddish color and at later stages turns it dirty reddish-brown. A dirty gray-greenish color results from hydrogen sulfide released during protein putrefaction, which transforms hemoglobin into sulfhemoglobin or verdoglobin. The metabolites of anaerobic bacteria are exclusively responsible for the strong odor of pus. They are also responsible for its putrid consistency.

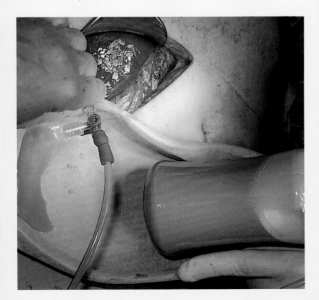

Pus drained from a liver abscess (before CT-guided drainage was available).

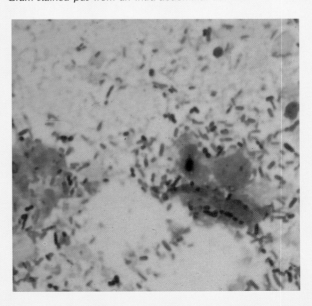

Gram-stained pus from an intra-abdominal abscess.

Causes of Infection

Perforation peritonitis is the most common form of acute intra-abdominal infection. In major hospitals, about 80% of cases are due to a variety of necrotic lesions of the gastrointestinal tract and other intra-abdominal organs; perforation is found in the stomach and duodenum in 31%, in the appendix in 22%, in the large bowel in 21%, and in the small bowel in 13%. All other origins of infection represent less than 9%.

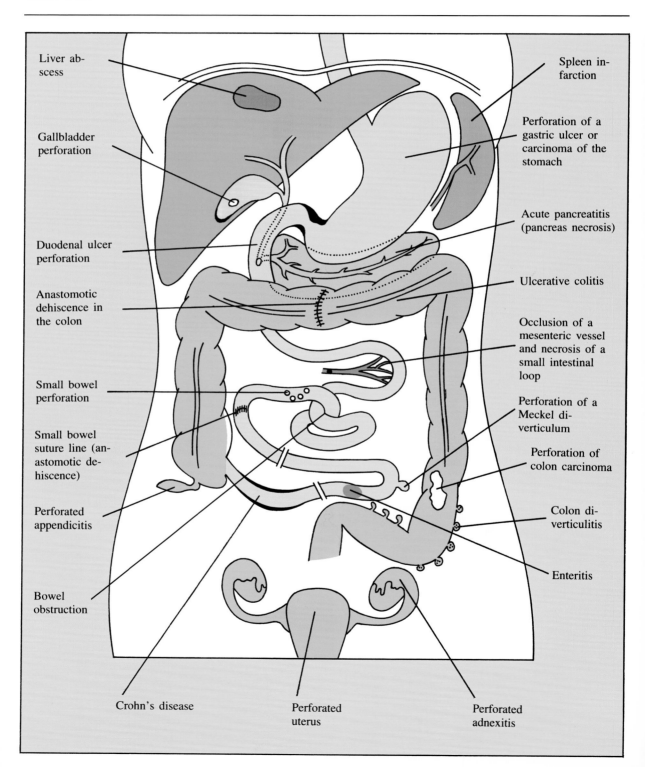

Liver abscess

Gallbladder perforation

Duodenal ulcer perforation

Anastomotic dehiscence in the colon

Small bowel perforation

Small bowel suture line (anastomotic dehiscence)

Perforated appendicitis

Bowel obstruction

Spleen infarction

Perforation of a gastric ulcer or carcinoma of the stomach

Acute pancreatitis (pancreas necrosis)

Ulcerative colitis

Occlusion of a mesenteric vessel and necrosis of a small intestinal loop

Perforation of a Meckel diverticulum

Perforation of colon carcinoma

Colon diverticulitis

Enteritis

Crohn's disease

Perforated uterus

Perforated adnexitis

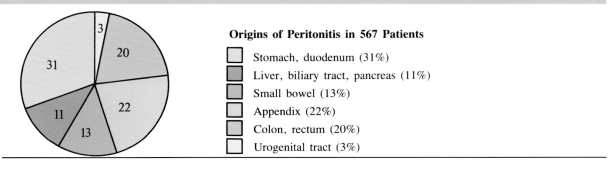

Origins of Peritonitis in 567 Patients

- ☐ Stomach, duodenum (31%)
- ☐ Liver, biliary tract, pancreas (11%)
- ☐ Small bowel (13%)
- ☐ Appendix (22%)
- ☐ Colon, rectum (20%)
- ☐ Urogenital tract (3%)

Bacterial Count in the Gastrointestinal Tract

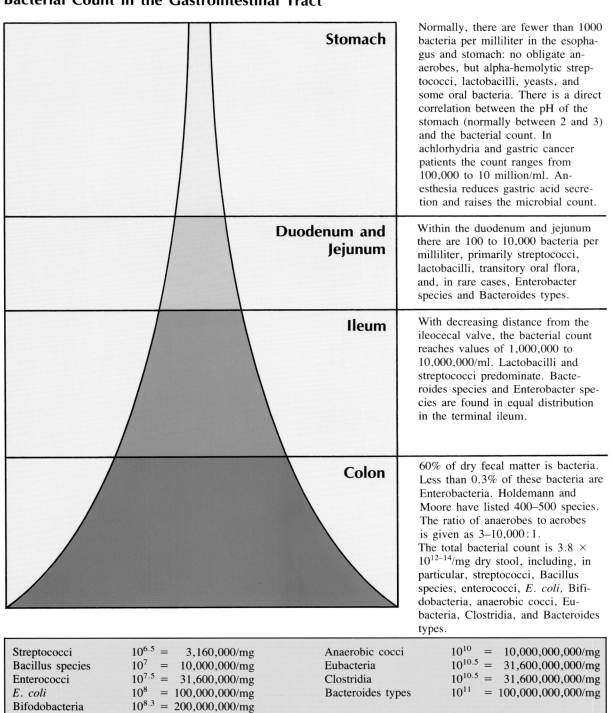

Stomach

Normally, there are fewer than 1000 bacteria per milliliter in the esophagus and stomach: no obligate anaerobes, but alpha-hemolytic streptococci, lactobacilli, yeasts, and some oral bacteria. There is a direct correlation between the pH of the stomach (normally between 2 and 3) and the bacterial count. In achlorhydria and gastric cancer patients the count ranges from 100,000 to 10 million/ml. Anesthesia reduces gastric acid secretion and raises the microbial count.

Duodenum and Jejunum

Within the duodenum and jejunum there are 100 to 10,000 bacteria per milliliter, primarily streptococci, lactobacilli, transitory oral flora, and, in rare cases, Enterobacter species and Bacteroides types.

Ileum

With decreasing distance from the ileocecal valve, the bacterial count reaches values of 1,000,000 to 10,000,000/ml. Lactobacilli and streptococci predominate. Bacteroides species and Enterobacter species are found in equal distribution in the terminal ileum.

Colon

60% of dry fecal matter is bacteria. Less than 0.3% of these bacteria are Enterobacteria. Holdemann and Moore have listed 400–500 species. The ratio of anaerobes to aerobes is given as 3–10,000:1.
The total bacterial count is $3.8 \times 10^{12-14}$/mg dry stool, including, in particular, streptococci, Bacillus species, enterococci, *E. coli,* Bifidobacteria, anaerobic cocci, Eubacteria, Clostridia, and Bacteroides types.

Streptococci	$10^{6.5}$	=	3,160,000/mg		
Bacillus species	10^{7}	=	10,000,000/mg		
Enterococci	$10^{7.5}$	=	31,600,000/mg		
E. coli	10^{8}	=	100,000,000/mg		
Bifodobacteria	$10^{8.3}$	=	200,000,000/mg		
Anaerobic cocci				10^{10} =	10,000,000,000/mg
Eubacteria				$10^{10.5}$ =	31,600,000,000/mg
Clostridia				$10^{10.5}$ =	31,600,000,000/mg
Bacteroides types				10^{11} =	100,000,000,000/mg

A rational therapy of intra-abdominal infections requires not only knowledge of pathology and anatomy of the disease, but also understanding of the biological properties of the pathogens. The bacteriological findings must be evaluated according to the pathogenic diversity.

Normal Bowel Flora

The pathogens of peritonitis stem primarily from the intestines and bordering hollow organs. Knowledge of types and frequency of bacteria in the various segments of the bowels provides the surgeon with the most probable etiology of the infection before bacteriological findings are available.

It must be borne in mind that the types of intestinal flora are determined by a patient's age, race, diet, previous operations, nutritional status, gastric acid, bile salts, gut motility, immunological mechanisms, prior administration of antibiotics, and other factors. It is therefore an oversimplification to speak of a blind or empiric initial antibiotic therapy. To be more precise, we should speak of a partially calculated antibiotic strategy.

Pathogens

Like all medically important bacteria, intra-abdominal pathogens are heterotrophic. These bacteria utilize organic material as a source of carbon and satisfy their energy requirements for the synthesis of cell components with the help of various enzyme-dependent metabolic pathways. Under optimal conditions these bacteria multiply rapidly by cell division every 20–30 minutes. Overall bacterial growth progresses in phases: A buildup phase dependent on environmental conditions and temperature is followed by an exponential phase of multiplication during which division rates reach a maximum as the bacterial population density increases. This growth phase ceases due to a depletion of

nutrients and an accumulation of toxic metabolites as well as the presence of host defenses with phagocytosis and autolysis. Outside the intestines only those bacteria that can withstand the body's defense system survive for any length of time. The pathogenicity, i.e., the virulence of a bacterium, can vary considerably within the same species. Bacteria can cause disease symptoms either directly (endotoxins, exotoxins, and others) or indirectly, by activation of host defenses. Different bacterial species can be characterized accordingly. Information on the pathogenicity of individual species is particularly important in mixed infections because the available therapeutics are not equally active against all pathogens. Hence, the choice of a therapeutic agent depends on those properties of individual bacteria that cause diseases.

Antibiotic therapy should begin immediately after sampling pus for bacteriological investigation; i.e., it should begin when the diagnosis has been confirmed by the operation. Antibiotic therapy should not be delayed by time-consuming identification of pathogens and sensitivity testing, since the explosive multiplication of pathogens, even following surgical treatment, can endanger the life of the patient.

However, such administration of antibiotics should not be blind; it must be well calculated. The antibiotics administered are directed against the defined target pathogens of intra-abdominal infections (see p. 69).

The isolation of pathogens poses many problems during routine work in hospitals. Many pathogens die rapidly after sampling and cannot be cultivated by the bacteriologist. A subsequent therapy will fail if it is based on bacteriological results gained under these conditions.

According to their origin, intra-abdominal infections are caused by a typical bacterial spectrum. Initially chemotherapy is directed against this spectrum. Nevertheless, pathogens must be identified individually. Bacteriological findings become significant should the initial antibiotic regimen show no success by the third day of treatment. Then, one can specifically address those microorganisms that the initial chemotherapy spared and, more important, that are responsible for the persistence of symptoms.

The identification of pathogens is a problem for the surgeon, since intra-abdominal infections are caused, in part, by bacteria difficult to cultivate. Often, surgery must be performed when the bacteriologist is not in a position to adequately handle the infectious material. Many bacteria die after only a brief exposure to oxygen and thus cannot be cultivated. In many cases the cultures reveal enterococci that are only weakly pathogenic but highly transport-resistant. Other pathogenic microorganisms responsible for a given infection will have already died during sampling transportation. A specific antibacterial therapy based on such isolation procedures would be doomed to failure. Although ampicillin, for example, is highly active against enterococci, it does not affect most of the bacteria that typically cause intra-abdominal infections.

Collection of Pathological Samples and Transportation

Immediately after the abdominal cavity has been opened, two plastic syringes are used to take up 10 ml each of pus free of air. (If air bubbles are present, they must be ejected into a swab saturated with alcohol.) If a bacteriologist cannot further handle the sample within the next 10 minutes, the pus and tissue must be spread out on at least five culture media. The plates can be placed in a gaspack system for anaerobic cultivation and hermetically closed. Further processing is carried out on the next day. The pus in the second syringe can be used for Gram-staining. In the absence of a gaspack system, small glass flasks in which air has been replaced with carbon dioxide can be used as a transport system. However, it should be borne in mind that all transport systems select bacteria. The frequently used thioglycolate medium, for example, selects *E. coli* and enterococci. As a rule, aerobes will survive transportation in an oxygen-free environment together with anaerobes. Still, separate transportation is preferable in order to register true aerobes such as *Pseudomonas aeruginosa*.

Gram-Staining

Infectious material from intra-abdominal infections can be Gram-stained during the course of surgery. This allows for the detection of atypical pathogens, type by type or in combination. Nevertheless, the results of Gram-staining are of limited value in a clinical setting. Gram-staining allows only for confirmation of the subsequent culture results. As a rule, Gram-staining reveals the typical picture of a mixed infection stemming from gram-positive and gram-negative cocci and rods; it does not permit a differentiated bacterial diagnosis.

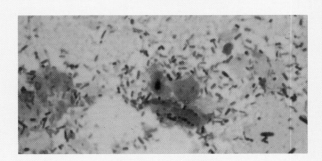

Sample of pus and necrotizing material taken after incision and immediately Gram-stained. As shown here, a structure comprising virtually all human pathogenic bacteria is typical for intra-abdominal infections.

Bacteria are microscopic organisms capable of biosynthesis and energy-producing reactions that support independent growth. They multiply through reduplication. Bacteria are prokaryotic organisms since they lack a true nucleus with a nuclear membrane, chromosomes, and a cellular apparatus for mitosis.

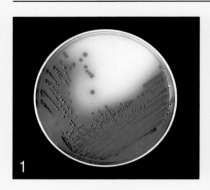

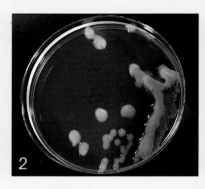

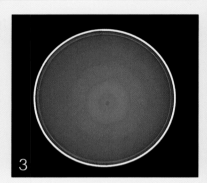

E. coli (Fig. 1)

Escherichia coli is a gram-negative, motile, rod-shaped bacterium. In terms of the frequency of bacteria in the large bowels, *E. coli* occupies positions 76 to 113. It accounts for 0.06% of total bacterial mass. 10^8 *E. coli* are found per milliliter of feces. Its relative share among all pathogens for intra-abdominal infections is 300 times greater than its relative share among all intestinal bacteria. This is an expression of its extraordinary pathogenicity. In animal experiments, *E. coli* is isolated in blood cultures during the septic phase of peritonitis in ~90% of all cases. Not all recognizable strains are pathogenic.

The negatively charged capsule of *E. coli* can resist phagocytosis. This is recognized as a factor contributing to its virulence. The capsule consists of polysaccharides (K-antigen). Motile flagella represent the H-antigen. Motility structures as well as the ability to adhere to cells are further parameters of pathogenicity. Specific lipopolysaccharides of the capsules are called O-antigens or endotoxins (see p. 36). In addition, extracellular products as well as proteolytic enzymes and exoenzymes destructive to the tissue have been described as virulence factors.

Klebsiella (Fig. 2)

Klebsiella are plump, nonflagellat-ed, encapsulated, gram-negative bacilli. They are less frequent in the colon than *E. coli*. In only 10% of the normal population can they be isolated from the bowels. As reflects their relative pathogenicity, Klebsiella are isolated ~50 times more frequently in peritoneal infections than in their natural environment in the feces. Klebsiella produce a highly active endotoxin (septic shock). They can be isolated in blood cultures. Furthermore, Klebsiella are often selected by treatment with newer broad-spectrum penicillins. Klebsiella also produce a beta-lactamase that is highly active against the old and new broad-spectrum penicillins.

Enterobacter species

Of clinical importance are *Enterobacter cloacae* and *Enterobacter aerogenes*. These microorganisms are facultative pathogenic and occur less frequently than Klebsiella in the bowels. As members of the Enterobacteriaceae family they, in part, exhibit pathogenic characteristics. However, in clinical circumstances they are less aggressive than *E. coli* and Klebsiella. Most antibiotics are not effective against Enterobacter species. These pathogens are often isolated during the second stage of infection when the clinical signs of the infection are receding. This observation points to their degree of pathogenicity. In extremely immunosuppressed patients, however, these organisms can cause therapeutic problems after other bacteria have already been eliminated. The relative occurrence of Enterobacter species in the bowels is 0.02%, in intra-abdominal infections 3.8%.

Proteus species (Fig. 3)

The genus Proteus comprises gram-negative rods. We mainly find the following four species as pathogens: the indole-nonfermenting *Proteus mirabilis* and the three indole-positive species *P. vulgaris, P. rettgeriand*, and *P. morganii*. All these species form spreading colonies on most agar plates (see photo). Their frequency in the bowels is less than 0.02%; in intra-abdominal infections their incidence is 6.9%.

Many species possess pili and can thus attach themselves to peritoneal cells. Flagella allow for motility and also heighten their virulence. The indole-positive strains are resistant against many antibiotics. Next to obligate anaerobic bacteria, *P. mirabilis* is very often isolated from abscesses. This species is highly pathogenic. This fact has been camouflaged during the past decades since most antibiotics, except for the newest ones, are active against this microorganism.

Aerobic bacteria multiply in the presence of oxygen. Most aerobes, however, are also facultative anaerobes; i.e., they multiply without oxygen. There is no satisfactory classification system of bacteria. The nomenclature in this text is based on *Bergey's Manual of Determinative Bacteriology.*

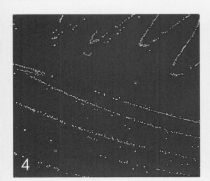

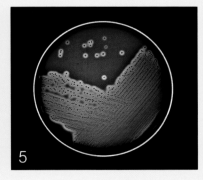

Enterococcus faecalis
(Fig. 4)

Enterococci are gram-positive, chain-forming cocci. Included in this group are various group D streptococci (*Enterococcus faecalis, E. faecium,* and *E. durans*). Their pathogenicity in intra-abdominal infections is low. Essentially, they contribute to the virulence of such anaerobic bacteria as *Bacteroides fragilis* and *Fusobacterium varium.* The frequency of enterococci in the bowels is 0.13%. Their frequency in intra-abdominal infections, always in combination with other bacteria, is 6.3%. They are highly resistant to transport and can frequently be isolated in bacteriological investigations long after other more sensitive anaerobic bacteria have died.

Enterococci are resistant against all aminoglycosides and most cephalosporins. They are selected by therapy with cephalosporins. They can frequently be isolated toward the final stages of intra-abdominal infections when they no longer provoke new symptoms of infection.

Other Streptococci (Fig. 5)

In intra-abdominal infections other streptococci, primarily those in group A and B, are isolated to a lesser degree (3.8%). With regard to their pathogenicity, cellular surface components and extracellular

components play an important role. The M-protein is antiphagocytic and suppresses opsonization. The hyaluronic acid capsule also acts antiphagocytically. The peptidoglycone has endotoxin properties and reduces the necrotic-purulent lesions. The lipo-teichoic acid enhances the adhesion to epithelial cells. Proteinases such as streptolysins O and S are cytotoxic; hyaluronidase and streptokinase promote the spread of infection. A pyrogenic exotoxin has endotoxinlike characteristics.

Staphylococci (Fig. 6)

Staphylococci are gram-positive cluster-forming cocci. As a pathogen in intra-abdominal infections, they occur only rarely (2.1%). Staphylococci are seldom found in the bowels. *Staphylococcus aureus* is an extracellular parasite. Thanks to a component in the cell wall (protein A), virulent species

withstand phagocytosis. In fact, this protein even prevents phagocytosis of opsonized staphylococci. Staphylococci produce a catalase that inhibits the intracellular killing by macrophages. Staphylococci also produce a glycocalyx, a pathogenic factor that is seldom recognized.

Pseudomonas aeruginosa
(Fig. 7)

Pseudomonas aeruginosa is a gram-negative nonfermenting rod. It belongs to a taxonomically mixed group of bacilli that have two important characteristics:
1. They cannot ferment carbohydrates.
2. They multiply only under aerobic conditions.

Their pathogenicity is significant in pulmonary infections, but they play a minor role as causative agents in intra-abdominal infections. Their frequency in the bowels is lower than 0.02%. Their share in causing intra-abdominal infections is 1.8%. Their extracellular products are considered important virulence factors: Exotoxin A is a potent inhibitor of protein synthesis and resembles diphtheria toxin. A number of pathogenic organisms produce potent lytic enzymes such as elastases and lecithinases.

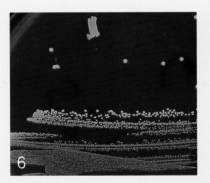

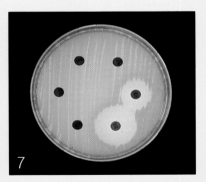

Anaerobic Bacteria

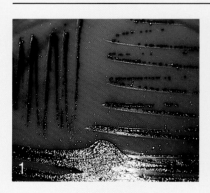

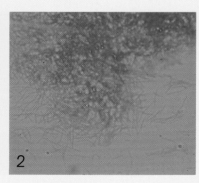

Bacteroides species
(Fig. 1)
Fusobacteria (Fig. 2)

Bacteroides species and Fusobacteria are gram-negative, pathogenic, non-spore-forming, rod-shaped bacteria. They occur in large numbers in the mouth, the intestines, and the female genital tract. They are strictly anaerobic and produce putrid odors and gas. Many species grow rather slowly; therefore their cultivation in the laboratory requires a week or longer before they can be identified.

The entire Bacteroides group is pleomorphic. *Bacteroides fragilis* is a nonfilamentous microorganism. It is difficult to distinguish *B. fragilis* morphologically from *E. coli,* as both organisms almost always appear together under normal circumstances. *Bacteroides fragilis* is the most important pathogen in the Bacteroides group. *Bacteroides melaninogenicus,* another highly pathogenic organism in this group, is frequently found in mixed cultures with other anaerobic bacteria. It produces growth factors for other bacteria. Infections stemming from Bacteroides species promote thrombophlebitis and septic embolism in the liver and other organs. Using proper techniques, Bacteroides species can be seen in >10% of all blood cultures.

The anaerobic rod-shaped bacteria produce exotoxins: *Fusobacterium necroforum* forms a leukocidin, *B. melaninogenicus* a collagenase. Other species produce neuraminidases. A heparinase produced by *B. fragilis* leads to intravascular coagulation and requires therapeutic augmentation of the heparin dose. *Bacteroides asaccharolyticus* shows a pronounced proteolytic ability, leading to the hydrolysis of collagenases, casein, and other lysed proteins. *Bacteroides melaninogenicus* and *B. intermedius* produce a lipase. All strains of the *B. fragilis* group, with the exception of *B. vulgatus,* release extracellular hyaluronidases and chondroitic sulfatases. Additionally, fibrolysin, lysosomal enzymes, lecithinases, desoxyribo-nucleases, phosphatases, proteinases, and lipases are produced by many Bacteroides species. Elastases are seldom found in this group. The endotoxin of Bacteroides species has shown low biological activity in most laboratory tests. *Bacteroides melaninogenicus* endotoxin contains no 2-keto-3-desoxy-octonate and no heptose. On the other hand, the endotoxins of *Fusobacterium necroforum* and *F. nucleatum* show a more pronounced biological activity comparable to that of *Salmonella enteritidis.*

In animal experiments, abscesses are difficult to produce by monocultures of these anaerobic bacteria. In order to form full-blown abscesses, other anaerobic bacteria are required.

Bacteroides species are the most frequently found microorganisms in the intestines. They account for 26% of the bowel flora. The prevalence of *B. fragilis* is 0.6%. However, it is found in 12% of all intra-abdominal infections, reflecting its pathogenicity.

The share of Fusobacteria in the normal intestinal flora is 7%, their relative frequency in infections 3.1%.

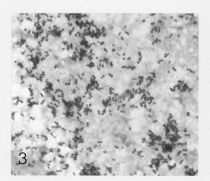

Peptostreptococci (Fig. 3)

Peptococci and peptostreptococci are gram-positive anaerobic cocci forming clusters and chains, respectively. They produce foul, putrid odors and gas. Normally, they are present in the colon, in the vagina, and in the oral cavity. Their relative frequency in the intestinal flora is 9.3%. They are involved in 6.9% of all intra-abdominal infections. Their pathogenicity is comparable to that of aerobic gram-positive cluster-forming and chain-forming cocci.

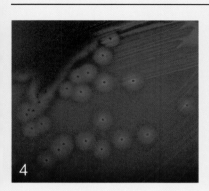

4

Clostridiae (Fig. 4)

Clostridiae are the only anaerobic gram-positive pathogens that form spores. Most pathogenic species do not form spores in the tissue. Although most Clostridiae are obligate anaerobes, two species (*Clostridium tertium* and *C. histolyticum*) can multiply aerobically. *Clostridium perfringens* is also aerotolerant. Hence, it is detected relatively frequently even when poor anaerobic isolation techniques are used.

Fewer than 10 of the 100 different Clostridiae species occurring in the bowels (5.9%) are pathogenic (0.7%). Clostridiae produce exotoxins leading to gas gangrene and botulism. Other Clostridiae, such as *C. perfringens, C. novyi,* and *C. septicum* as well as the rare species *C. histolyticum, C. bifermentans,* and *C. fallax,* produce myonecroses, anaerobic phlegmon, septic abortions, and severe intra-abdominal and wound infections. The toxin of *C. difficile* induces a pseudomembranous colitis.

Clostridiae are the most virulent anaerobes. Their exotoxins lead to fulminant tissue destruction and rapid death of the host. The lecithinases of *C. perfringens* (alphatoxin) and *C. novyi* (gammatoxin) destroy cell membranes. Liquids and proteins can permeate the cellular walls and lead to a total destruction of the tissue. The alphatoxin of *C. perfringens* is capable of lysing red blood corpuscles. As a rule, this leads to hemolytic anemia and hemoglobinuria, typical consequences of the sepsis provoked by these microorganisms. The collagenases of *C. perfringens* and *C. histolyticum* destroy all collagen barriers in the tissue and thus undermine localization of the infection by host defenses. The destruction of capillary-bound reticulins leads to bleeding and thrombosis and ultimately to a reduction of redox potential. In addition, the growth of these organisms is encouraged by proteolysis due to recrudescence of amino acids and peptides. The hyaluronidase of *C. perfringens* facilitates the rapid propagation of this microorganism to other tissues. Other important pathogenic exoenzymes are desoxyribonucleases (*C. perfringens* and *C. septicum*), lipases *(C. novyi),* proteinases *(C. histolyticum),* and fibrolysins. Furthermore, these organisms produce hemolysins, neuraminidases, phospholipases, lysolecithins, elastases, and leukocidins.

Propionibacteria (Fig. 5)

The anaerobic diphtheroid *Corynebacterium acnes* (synonym *Propionibacterium acnes*) is the most frequent skin organism in humans. It is isolated in mixed infections. Its pathogenic significance is low. Its relative frequency of occurrence in the bowels is 0.2%. It is seen in 3.1% of the cases in intra-abdominal infections. However, it always occurs in combination with other pathogenic anaerobic bacteria.

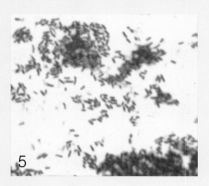

5

Veillonella cocci (Fig. 6)

Veillonella are the most common gram-negative anaerobic micrococci in humans. They are strictly anaerobic and normally occur in the oral cavity, the upper respiratory

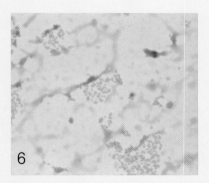

6

tract, the vagina, and the intestinal tract (frequency 0.2%). Their pathogenicity is not well researched. In intra-abdominal infections they are isolated in 1.4% of cases. Furthermore, they are isolated in abscesses and pulmonary infections, mostly in combination with other anaerobic bacteria.

27

Of the myriad microorganisms in the intestines, only a few are capable of causing infections in humans, and even fewer can precipitate surgical infections.

As a source of pathogens, the gastrointestinal tract contains under normal conditions a high bacterial count of $10^{12-14}/$ml. This number represents about 400 different bacteria species. Their quantitative and qualitative distribution depends on functional status and prior damage. From this bacterial mass few pathogenic bacteria are selected following perforation and migration, since most organisms in the intestinal flora cannot exist outside their natural environment. This is especially true of obligate anaerobic bacteria, whose frequency in the intestines is more than 1000 times greater than that of aerobic microorganisms. Nonetheless, the relative frequency of obligate anaerobes is low in intra-abdominal infections.

As soon as bacteria reach the peritoneal cavity via the necrotic hollow organ wall, the metabolic balance regulating saprophytic, symbiotic, and parasitic functions is disturbed. Initially, the body's peritoneal defense mechanism in the peritoneal cavity also disturbs the intraluminary balance. As a result, pathogenic bacteria multiply unproportionally. Empirically, the pathogenicity of individual bacterial species is expressed as the ratio of their frequency in infections to their frequency in intraluminary occurrences.

The Most Common Pathogens of Intra-abdominal Infections

Aerobes*	Gram-negative	E. coli	Rods
		Klebsiella spp.	
		Enterobacter spp.	
		Proteus spp.	
		Pseudomonas aeruginosa	
	Gram-positive	Enterococci	Cocci
		Other streptococci	
		Staphylococcus aureus	
		Other bacteria and yeasts	
Anaerobes†	Gram-negative	Bacteroides fragilis	Rods
		Other Bacteroides spp.	
		Fusobacterium spp.	
		Veillonella spp.	Cocci
	Gram-positive	Propionibacterium spp.	Cocci
		Peptococcus spp.	
		Peptostreptococcus spp.	
		Clostridium spp.	Rods

*Also facultative anaerobes except Pseudomonas.
†Obligate anaerobes.

Relative Frequency of Pathogens in the Colon			
E. coli	0.06%	Total aer. 0.31%	
Klebsiella spp.	0.03%		
Enterobacter spp.	0.02%		
Proteus spp.	0.02%		
	0.13%		
Pseudomonas aeruginosa	<0.02%		Other bacteria and yeasts (non-pathogenic) to 100%
Enterococci	0.13%		
Other streptococci	0.02%		
Staphylococcus aureus	0.01%		
	0.18%		
Total aerobes	0.31%		
Bacteroides fragilis	0.6%		
Other Bacteroides	26.0%		
Fusobacterium spp.	7.0%		
Veillonella spp. 0.2% Propionibacterium spp. 0.2%	0.4%		
Peptococcus spp.	9.3%		
Peptostreptococcus spp.	12.0%		
Clostridium spp.	0.7%		

Relative Occurrence of Pathogens in 900 Intra-abdominal Infections (Perforation)		
E. coli	51%	87%
Klebsiella spp.	14%	
Enterobacter spp.	6%	
Proteus spp.	16%	
Pseudomonas spp.	7%	49%
Enterococci	17%	
Other streptococci	12%	
Staphylococci	5%	
Other aerobes	8%	
Bacteroides fragilis	37%	72%
Other Bacteroides	35%	
Fusobacterium spp.	7%	14%
Veillonella spp.	2%	
Propionibacterium spp.	5%	
Peptococcus spp.	8%	21%
Peptostreptococcus spp.	13%	
Clostridium spp.	23%	23%
Other anaerobes	21%	21%

The Qualitative Pathogenicity of Causative Agents

The synergistic pathogenicity of causative agents involved in intra-abdominal infections can be clearly observed in animal experiments. The clinical progression of the disease in the absence of therapeutic measures corresponds well with experimental findings.

Weinstein and Onderdonk implanted cecal feces mixed with barium sulfate in the free peritoneal cavity. They thereby showed a reproducible biphasic disease, similar to the natural course of intra-abdominal infections.

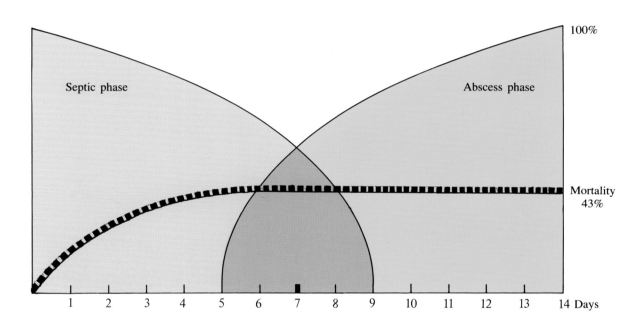

The initial septic phase of peritonitis lasts from the first to about the seventh day of infection. An abscess stage develops by the fifth day. During the septic-peritonitic phase, *E. coli* is observed in most blood cultures. Given a defined inoculum size, 39% of the animals died during the first phase. The surviving animals develop abscesses in which Bacteroides species and Fusobacteria are more frequent than enterococci and *E. coli*.

These experiments raise the following question: Can both phases of intra-abdominal infection be reproduced by inoculation of single bacterial species? To answer this question, monocultures and defined combinations of bacteria were inoculated together with barium sulfate. The results of these experiments reveal the significance of individual bacterial species relative to the phases of intra-abdominal infections.

Recent investigations have reproduced the picture of intra-abdominal infection with initial septic and protracted abscess phases, using only the endotoxin of *E. coli* and the capsule of *Bacteroides fragilis.*

Experiments

1) Monocultures of *E. coli*

Intraperitoneal inoculation with $10^{7.3}$ of *E. coli* leads to the septic phase of peritonitis only, with a mortality of 30%. No abscess phase is observed in survivors.

2) Monocultures of *Bacteroides fragilis* and Fusobacteria

Intraperitoneal inoculation of $10^{7.8}$ of either *B. fragilis* or *F. varium* yield no mortality or abscesses. These anaerobes in monoculture are obviously of little pathogenicity in this model.

3) Monocultures of *Enterococcus faecalis*

Intraperitoneal inoculation of high counts of *Enterococcus faecalis* (four times the quantity in the *E. coli* experiment) did not result in peritonitis. No mortality and no abscess formation were seen, indicating that this organism alone is also of low pathogenicity.

4) Mixed Cultures of *E. coli* and Bacteroides

Intraperitoneal inoculation of $10^{7.3}$ *E. coli* (as in the first experiment) combined with $10^{7.8}$ of *Bacteroides fragilis* leads to the typical full-blown biphasic picture of intra-abdominal infection. In the septic peritonitic phase 43% die. Abscesses were observed in all surviving animals.

5) *Enterococcus faecalis* and *Bacteroides fragilis*

Whereas high inocula of both *Bacteroides fragilis* alone and *Enterococcus faecalis* alone do not induce sepsis or abscesses, the combination of the two induces a full abscess phase. In other words, to form abscesses *Bacteroides fragilis* is dependent on aerobic pathogens such as *Enterococcus faecalis*, which alone, as noted above, does not elicit the disease in this model. No septic/peritonitis phase, however, is seen with this combination.

The importance of bacterial adherence is shown in the electron microscopic figures below. Little is known about what influences bacterial adherence to the peritoneum.

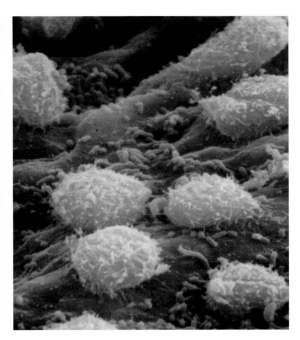

Biopsy from serosal mesothelium 24 hours after cecal ligation and puncture (diffuse peritonitis model) demonstrating inflammatory cells and bacteria on the peritoneal mesothelium (5000×). (Courtesy of Dr. C. E. Edmiston.)

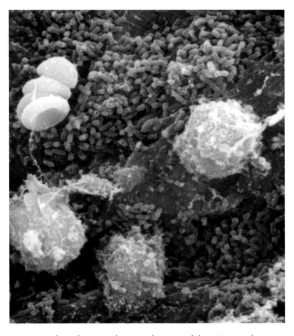

Peritoneal surface 24 hours after cecal ligation and puncture (diffuse peritonitis) reveals dense microbial colonization of the mesothelium and numerous macrophages and other blood constituents (RBCs) (5000×). (Courtesy of Dr. C. E. Edmiston.)

Peritonitis represents the inflammatory reaction of peritoneal tissue elicited by chemical and physical noxae. Bacteria and their toxins play a key role as causative agents. The local tissue lesions trigger the influx of bacteria-containing gastrointestinal content into the abdominal cavity. Immediately after the influx of bacteria into the free peritoneal cavity— mostly after intestinal necrosis— these bacteria multiply, depending on their adaptability to the new environment. The damage caused by these events takes the course described below.

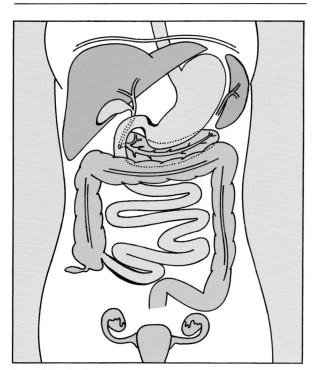

Intra-abdominal organs.

1. Histamine and other vasoactive substances are released due to mast cell degranulation following cell damage to the peritoneum.

2. Conversely, complements are activated and chemotaxis is induced.

3. Vasoactive substances increase the permeability of vessels. In combination with chemotaxis, this promotes the influx of polymorphonuclear granulocytes. The latter, along with local macrophages, phagocytize bacteria. This process is supported by the activation of complements, which, in turn, is initiated by opsonization. Finally, phagocytized bacteria are destroyed and carried away.

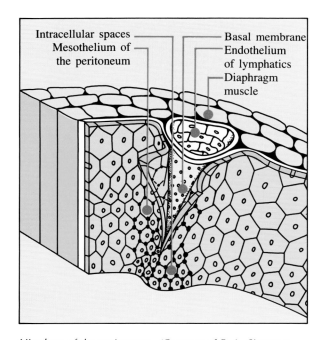

Histology of the peritoneum. (Courtesy of R. L. Simmons, The Upjohn Company, 1981.)

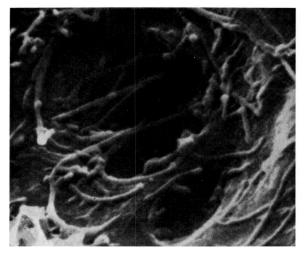

REM picture of peritoneal stoma from the diaphragm (4–12 µm). (Courtesy of E. C. Tsilibary, S. L. Wissig, Am J Anat 149:131, 1977.)

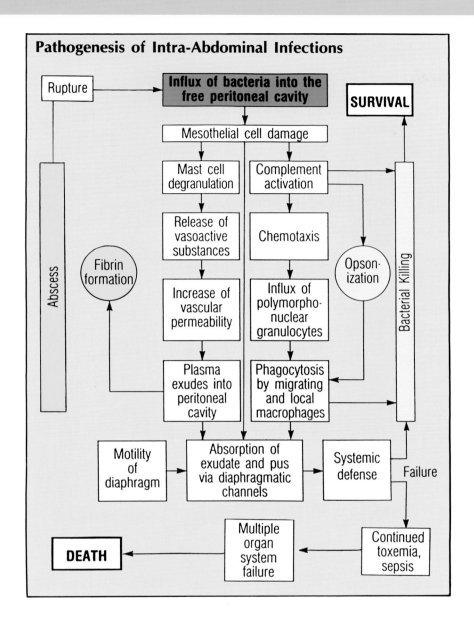

Pathogenesis of Intra-Abdominal Infections

Rupture → Influx of bacteria into the free peritoneal cavity

SURVIVAL

Mesothelial cell damage

Mast cell degranulation

Complement activation

Release of vasoactive substances

Chemotaxis

Fibrin formation

Opson- ization

Abscess

Increase of vascular permeability

Influx of polymorpho- nuclear granulocytes

Bacterial Killing

Plasma exudes into peritoneal cavity

Phagocytosis by migrating and local macrophages

Motility of diaphragm

Absorption of exudate and pus via diaphragmatic channels

Systemic defense

Failure

Multiple organ system failure

Continued toxemia, sepsis

DEATH

---

4. Due to the increased vascular permeability, plasma is exudated into the free peritoneal cavity, leading to fibrin formation. In this way, necrotic and bacteria-containing districts are demarked, leading to abscess formation.

5. On the other hand, absorption of exudate and pus through the diaphragmatic lymphatic channels also represents important defense mechanisms in the peritoneal cavity. This defense reaction is enhanced by respiratory motion in connection with the diaphragmatic lymphatic valves. 80% of the exudate and noxae are absorbed via thoratic lymph channels into the venous portion of the central circulatory system. Thus,

this material is subject to systemic defense mechanisms.

Adjuvants

Many experiments have demonstrated the infection-promoting effect of certain substances known as adjuvants.

Sterile stool, barium sulfate, bile, mucus and **hemoglobin** can, if inoculated, lead to a lethal peritonitis, although the bacterial count may be lower than usual in such cases. These substances strain the phagocytotic capacity of neutrophilic granulocytes, to the detriment of phagocytosis of the bacteria.

Hemoglobin: Hau was able to demonstrate that hemoglobin inhibited the intraperitoneal chemotaxis of neutrophilic granulocytes, the intracellular killing of bacteria, phagocytosis, and the transdiaphragmatic absorption of bacteria.

Iron ions and pigments are released by the breakdown of hemoglobin. These substances are considered to have toxic effects.

Bile per se is not toxic. However, it reduces surface tension and promotes the spreading of bacteria.

Mucus is said to inhibit phagocytosis by coating bacteria.

Given a high bacterial count with considerable amounts of noxious material and a rapid intra-abdominal clearance, intraperitoneal infections encroach upon the entire organism at an early stage. This can lead to damage to all organ systems. In effect, a local infection turns into a severe systemic infectious disease.

The inflammatory reaction of the peritoneum implicates a significant sequestration of fluid in the peritoneal cavity. The total surface area of the peritoneum measures 2 m^2, of which 1.0 to 1.4 m^2 represent functional tissue. The occurrence of an inflammatory edema expanding the peritoneum to a thickness of 5 mm results in a fluid loss of 5 to 8 L from the entire organism, i.e., from the circulation system to the peritoneal cavity. This leads to an initial hypovolemic shock, followed by dehydration and, finally, by the patient's death in connection with toxin-induced shock. Sepsis is due mainly to the products of bacterial breakdown.

Hypoxia forms the turnstile of all the pathophysiological mechanisms. It occurs as a result of septic-toxic circulatory insufficiency by a reduced supply of oxygen (respiratory insufficiency, reduced pulmonary oxygen transport, reduced nutritive perfusion), by reduced oxygen delivery to the tissue (increased O$_2$ affinity of hemoglobin), and by reduced oxygen utilization (due to endotoxin-inhibited ATP synthesis in the mitochondria).

Damage to Vital Organs

1. Heart

Dehydration, tachycardia, hypotension, reduction of circulation time and of cardiac output and venous return with increased peripheral resistance (blood pooling), hypoxia, shock. Endotoxin shock may follow, its hyperdynamic and subsequent hypodynamic pattern superposing preexisting shock forms.

2. Lung

Disturbance of pulmonary distribution with atrial venous shunting, increase in pulmonary resistance, alveolar cell destruction, increase of oxygen transfer distance, pulmonary insufficiency, hypoxia, shock lung, or acute respiratory distress syndrome. Atelectasis due to increased intra-abdominal pressure.

3. Kidney

Reduced perfusion in the presence of hypovolemia, increased intra-abdominal pressure and augmented buildup of toxic metabolites, hypoxic and toxic damage to renal epithelia, increase in urea nitrogen and creatinine, renal insufficiency.

4. Intestines

Local hypoxia, increased sympathetic activity, disproportionate bacterial growth, translocation, bowel distension, reduction of perfusion and influx of toxins into the circulation, increase of intra-abdominal pressure with negative effects on renal and pulmonary function.

Acute Respiratory Distress Syndrome

Acute respiratory distress syndrome (ARDS) develops in connection with interstitial and alveolary edema. The latter are brought about by plasma exudation with the disturbance of permeability of capillary membranes, by septic circulatory changes, and by coagulation disorders, as well as reduced functional residual capacity.

Pulmonary comorbidity, age, obesity, laparotomy, anesthesia, and increased abdominal pressure stemming from the infection have an unfavorable effect on functional residual capacity. ARDS is also seen after trauma without a septic cause. It is believed to be due to overwhelming host defense mechanisms.

The disturbance of oxygen supply, delivery, and utilization results in hypoxia, which is the turnstile of the pathophysiological mechanism.

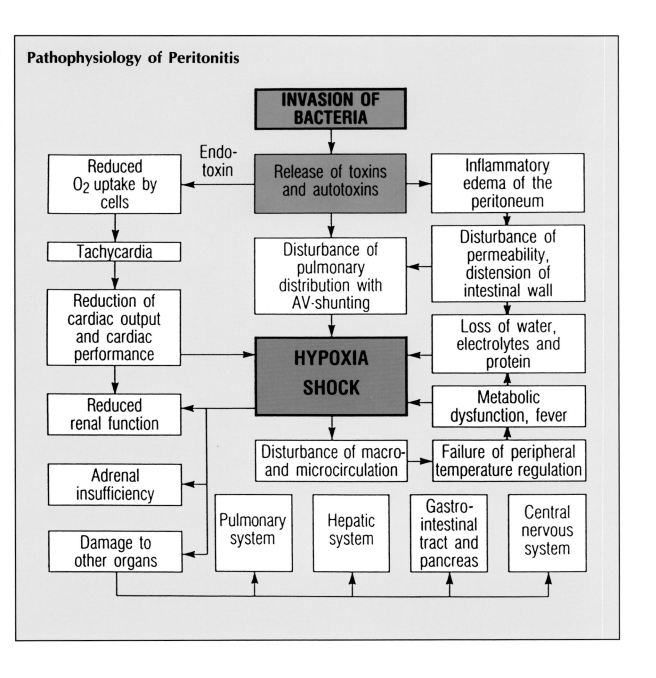

Pathophysiology of Peritonitis

INVASION OF BACTERIA

Endo-toxin

Release of toxins and autotoxins

Reduced O$_2$ uptake by cells

Inflammatory edema of the peritoneum

Tachycardia

Disturbance of pulmonary distribution with AV-shunting

Disturbance of permeability, distension of intestinal wall

Reduction of cardiac output and cardiac performance

Loss of water, electrolytes and protein

HYPOXIA SHOCK

Reduced renal function

Metabolic dysfunction, fever

Adrenal insufficiency

Disturbance of macro- and microcirculation

Failure of peripheral temperature regulation

Damage to other organs

Pulmonary system

Hepatic system

Gastro-intestinal tract and pancreas

Central nervous system

The Effect of IAI on the Entire Organism

1 ng endotoxin per kg body weight results in irreversible shock and death within 2 hours.

Endotoxins

Whereas most thermolabile exotoxins are released by living bacteria, thermostabile endotoxins are released during bacterial decay. Endotoxins are complex molecules of high molecular weight. They consist of phospholipids, polysaccharides, and proteins. These compounds form the outer cell wall of decomposed gram-positive bacteria and account for their toxic biological properties.

E. coli endotoxin:

Fs = Fatty acid

P = Phosphate

EtNH = Ethanol amine

KDO = 2-Keto-3- desoxyoctane acid

◯ = Sugar: glc = glucose

gal = galactose

hept = 1-glycero-D-mannoheptose

col = Colitose

(glc)(NH₂) = Glycosamine

(glc)NAc = N-Acetyl-glucosamine

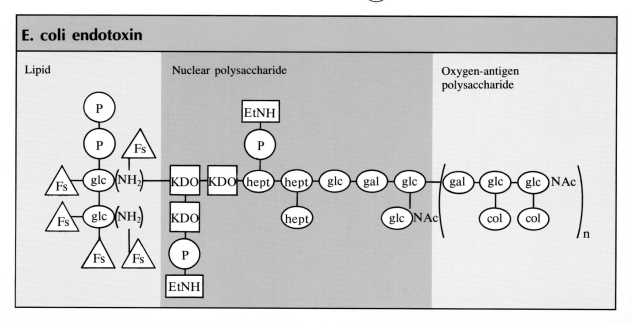

E. coli endotoxin

Lipid | Nuclear polysaccharide | Oxygen-antigen polysaccharide

36

Clinically measurable endotoxic effects are:

- Fever
- Increased vagotonus
- Leukopenia/leukocytosis

- Thrombopenia

- Consumptive coagulopathy (DIC)
- Hyper- and then hypoglycemia
- Increased plasma lipids and hepatic enzymes
- Reduced serum iron values

In Lower Doses Endotoxins Affect the Following Systems

Reticuloendothelial System (RES)

Mediators such as collagenases, pyrogenic prostaglandins, and coagulation factors are released from the macrophages via an over-reaction to cytotoxicity. Animal experiments show the reduction of the clearance of such compounds as colloidal carbon as a result of overwhelming reactions. After 7 days the RES is stimulated to produce antibodies against endotoxins.

Temperature-Regulation Center

Endotoxins act directly on the hypothalamus and cause fever. Furthermore, pyrogenic substances are released from neutrophilic granulocytes.

Blood

Endotoxins shift erythropoiesis from the bone marrow to the spleen. They cause leukopenia, followed by leukocytosis after 2–6 hours. In small doses, endotoxins increase phagocytotic activity and bacteria killing. Endotoxins produce an initial thrombopenia, accompanied by thrombocyte aggregation and lysis, so that ADP, vasoactive amines, histamine, serotonin, and platelet factor III are released. As a consequence of all these events, consumptive coagulopathy (DIC) is seen.

Coagulation

In the extrinsic system, endotoxins lead to a release of a tissue factor stemming from macrophages, of a platelet factor, and of thromboplastins. In the intrinsic system, factor XII (Hageman factor) is activated. This leads to disseminated intravascular coagulation in the sense of a localized and generalized Shwartzman-Sanarelli phenomenon. Additionally, vasoactive substances such as histamine, serotonin, and kinin are released into the vascular system.

Metabolic System

a) Initially, endotoxins induce hyperglycemia followed by hypoglycemia after several hours.
b) Endotoxins lead to hyperlipidemia and to a higher uptake of free fatty acids, cholesterins, phospholipids, and triglycerides.
c) Protein synthesis of the liver is stimulated; increasing amounts of lactate dehydrogenase (LDH), transaminases, and phosphokinases are released.

Other Effects

Endotoxins precipitate the increased release of adrenocorticotrophic hormone (ACTH), growth hormone (HGH), and cortisone; thyrotropin (TSH) and luteinizing hormone (LH) are influenced. Plasma iron levels and the total iron-binding capacity are reduced. A possible vagotonic effect results in decreased thirst and appetite, the stomach is emptied with delay, and diarrhea may occur. (In light of interactions stemming from intestinal paralysis due to peritonitis, the phenomenon clinicians refer to as *Reizstühle* becomes understandable.)

Septic Shock

Sudden overload of the organism with endotoxin leads to septic shock. During the initial hyperdynamic phase, this form of shock is explained by the inability of cells to utilize oxygen and the attempt by the circulatory system to compensate for this. The last stage is hypodynamic due to exhaustion.

Digression: The Clinical Picture of Peritonitis

Clinically, peritonitis presents itself as an "acute abdomen." The clinical picture varies according to the underlying disease, the topographical relationship to other intra-abdominal organs, the extent of damage to serous surfaces, and the status of host factors (for example, immunosuppression).

Case History

Anamnestic data may be decisive for the diagnostic and the localization of peritonitis. In many cases, peritonitis begins with a dull pain that cannot be localized. This visceral pain is transmitted via the solar plexus in the upper abdomen. This is initially coupled with nausea and vomiting. The later irritation of the parietal peritoneum is focused on the site of infection; the patient is usually in a position to indicate this clearly.

Other forms of peritonitis, e.g., after perforation of a peptic ulcer, develop suddenly in otherwise healthy patients. These patients experience severe pain due to irritation of the peritoneum. In all forms of peritonitis in which damage to the parietal peritoneum has occurred, patients indicate that the slightest movement increases pain. At first, voluntary immobilization of the peritoneal cavity is seen to reduce the pain. This is later replaced by reflectory spasms in the musculature encompassing the peritoneal cavity.

Physical Findings

The patient is dehydrated (dry tongue, sunken eyes), and the abdomen is tender. The localization of maximum pain and perforation may diverge. Rebound tenderness indicates irritation of the parietal peritoneum. If the patient is still able to suppress abdominal surface rigidity, the disease is in its early stage. As the disease progresses, reflectory abdominal rigidity due to muscular spasms occurs. This is a less favorable prognostic sign.

The initially excited and agitated patient becomes increasingly sedate. Breathing becomes flat because there is reduced diaphragmatic activity in order to alleviate pain. Anorexia, nausea, and vomiting in connection with reduced thirst are usually observed. Urinary output is diminished. Due to a paralytic ileus, the intestines are inflated and bowel sounds are reduced. There is fever and tachycardia. A rectal or vaginal investigation can point to a pathological lesion in this area when pain and fluctuation are observed. The physician must examine for a hidden hernial orifice.

Notes on the Case History

It is not advisable to rely solely on a patient's current complaints; the earlier medical history must be considered. If the patient has experienced a peptic ulcer in the past, peritonitis due to ulcer perforation is probable. A history of biliary stones can point not only to peritonitis but also to pancreatitis. A history of cardiovascular disease can point to ischemia of the intestines. Earlier operations point to an ileus and peritonitis due to necrotic bowel wall perforation. This is also true for incisional hernias. Inflammatory bowel disease is indicative of perforations in the corresponding bowel segment. Finally, peritonitis may be caused by iatrogenic manipulation or the use of other instruments, but these may be difficult to establish.

Laboratory Findings

In diffuse peritonitis there is an initial leukocytosis at a rate of 15,000/ml with a left shift, granulocytosis, and lymphopenia. In exceptionally severe cases, leukopenia can also be observed. Hematocrit and urea nitrogen readings are elevated. The acid-base balance is disturbed, and there is hypernatremia and hypokalemia. Aside from pancreatitis, amylase values can also be elevated in cases of an ileus and peptic ulcer. Where abdominal symptoms are only weakly pronounced and the disease progresses subacutely, an elevated erythrocyte sedimentation rate can be an important indicator. Blood cultures provide further evidence.

X-ray Findings

An x-ray of the thorax can show an elevation of the diaphragm and free air beneath the diaphragm pointing to a free perforation. In a general radiograph of the abdomen, a mechanical ileus can be differentiated from a paralytic ileus. Intestinal loops separated by liquid indicate increased exudation into the peritoneal cavity. A prominent psoas shadow is evidence of a retroperitoneal abscess. Pockets of air in the biliary tract make a biliary genesis of peritonitis probable. Occasionally, extraluminary levels are indicative of abscesses with anaerobic bacteria. Finally, basal atelectases and pleural infusions shown by chest x-ray can provide evidence for the underlying disease.

Special Forms of Peritonitis

Biliary Peritonitis

Sterile bile in the peritoneal cavity is called choleperitoneum, or cholascos. This alone does not produce peritonitis. Only the gradual growth of bacteria stemming from biliary tract infections may lead to peritonitis. Because these cases progress slowly, the diagnosis of peritonitis is often delayed. Therefore, in the past, peritonitis in connection with a biliary leak had an unfavorable prognosis.

Ulcer Perforation

At first, an ulcer perforation leads to chemical peritonitis. Its presentation is typical, and it is seldom misdiagnosed. An initial sharp pain accompanied by a rigid, scyphoid abdomen with free air under the diaphragm (in 80% of the cases) is pathognomonic. If the ulcer perforation is older than 12 hours, bacterial contamination is very likely. Chemical peritonitis due to ulcer perforation progresses to bacterial peritonitis. After 6 hours, bacteria can be isolated from the peritoneal cavity in 30% of the patients; after 24 hours, this is the case in all patients.

Pancreatitis

Initially, there is no bacterial inflammation. In later stages, however, intestinal paralysis is accompanied by bacterial migration and possibly translocation into the inflamed area, eventually resulting in bacterial peritonitis.

Ileus and Other Forms of Peritonitis

The causes of other forms of peritonitis are shown in the diagram on p. 20. Due to the obstructed clearance of intestinal content, there is increased intraluminary bacterial growth in the proximal segments of the intestines and accumulation of fluids and gas. These events, in turn, lead to an expansion of the intestinal walls and elongation of vessels, reducing oxygen and nutrient supply. The bowel wall suffers hypoxic damage, initiating the transmigration of intestinal bacteria into the free peritoneal cavity.

Intra-Abdominal Abscess

Intra-abdominal abscesses occur when host defense localizes influxing bacteria by producing a fibrin capsule around the lesion. Usually, this requires 10^7 bacteria per milliliter plus additional factors.

Intra-abdominal abscesses occur in solitary or multiple form. They consist of necrotic tissue, bacteria, and white cells. They are separated from the rest of the peritoneal cavity by fibrinous membranes. Most abscesses are formed at predestined anatomical sites. However, abscesses occur throughout the peritoneal cavity and even in parenchymatic organs. Abscesses are the result of various noxae, especially after the influx of intestinal bacterial masses through inflammatory perforation, intestinal ischemia, or trauma, or after operations. Abscesses are also formed after hematogenous dispersion (spleen), canalicular ascension (liver), or transmigration and translocation. As a rule, abscesses require 5 to 7 days to develop. Their clinical manifestation depends on the causes and the bacterial flora delivered by perforation.

The rupture of an abscess again initiates a diffuse intra-abdominal infection. The causative agents are now proliferating anaerobic microorganisms that have already become virulent.

Clinical Picture

The clinical presentation of an abscess depends on its anatomical localization. Case history and palpation findings are decisive indicators. The toxic signs of diffuse peritonitis are less pronounced. Ultrasound and computerized tomography have facilitated better diagnosis and nonoperative treatment.

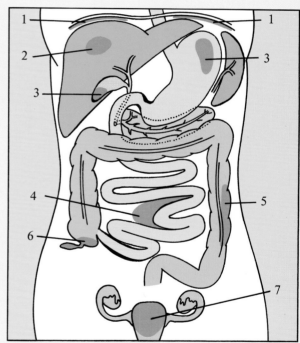

Location of abscesses
1 = Subphrenic   4 = Interenteric
2 = Hepatic   5 = Paracolic
3 = Subhepatic   6 = Pericecal
                     7 = Douglas

Diagnosis

Aside from physical examination, sonography, computer tomography, and, to a lesser degree, x-rays, help localize abscesses.

Bacterial Spectrum

The anaerobic bacteria predominantly found in intra-abdominal abscesses are usually isolated together with aerobic microorganisms. These aerobic and facultative anaerobic microorganisms are present in smaller numbers in abscesses.

Therapy

Intra-abdominal abscesses are classically treated by laparotomy and drained. Recently, there has been a positive trend toward extra-abdominal drainage of abscesses under ultrasound and computer-tomographic guidance.

Postoperative peritonitis is a dreaded complication of abdominal surgery due to breakdown of anastomoses and suture lines in entodermal organs. This form of peritonitis has a higher mortality than acute perforative peritonitis.

Clinical Picture

The clinical signs of postoperative peritonitis are often masked by postoperative physiological alterations of the organism and applied therapy. Pain, possible respiratory complications, paralysis, and fever can occur postoperatively in peritonitis with or without suture-line breakdown.

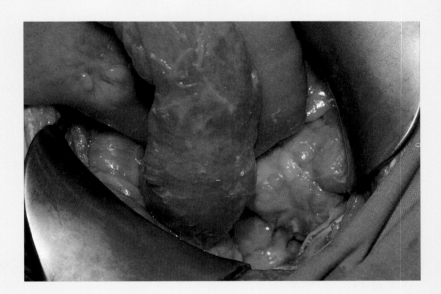

Peritonitis due to breakdown of the anastomotic suture line. The defective anastomosis is seen at lower right.

Diagnosis

Purulent secretion from drains may lead to the diagnosis. However, this material is often occluded and may be misinterpreted. The abdominal wound must be closely examined to detect purulent subfascial secretions. An x-ray in conjunction with a water-soluble contrast fluid can reveal a leak in the intestines. Palpation of the abdominal wall does not always yield reliable results. The concomitant application of analgesic medication can alter the patient's reaction to pain. Likewise, epidural anesthesia interferes with normal pain response.

Bacterial Spectrum

Bacteria isolated from postoperative peritonitis are altered by nosocomial influences. Hospital-based multi-resistant bacteria are often seen in this situation. They reflect the hospital's own antibiotic policy.

Therapy

The decisive measure in the treatment of postoperative peritonitis is the early operative revision of the peritoneal cavity and the complete elimination of the focus of infection. Given specific anatomical locations, this is often not possible, as in the case of suture-line breakdown after gastrectomy. In such cases, the mortality rate of intra-abdominal infections is high because the foci cannot be removed.

Since intra-abdominal infection takes many forms, there are a number of classification schemes. No classification is perfect. It is not possible to develop a practical classification system that would include all aspects of this disease, such as chemical peritonitis, intra-abdominal abscess, spontaneous peritonitis, traumatic peritonitis, serofibrinous peritonitis, etc.

Classification According to Etiology

I. **Primary peritonitis**
   A. Spontaneous peritonitis in children
   B. Spontaneous peritonitis in adults
   C. Peritonitis in patients with CAPD
   D. Tuberculous peritonitis
   E. Other forms

II. **Secondary peritonitis**
   A. Acute perforation peritonitis (acute suppurative peritonitis)
     1. GI tract perforation
     2. Bowel wall necrosis (intestinal ischemia)
     3. Pelviperitonitis
     4. Other forms
   B. Postoperative peritonitis
     1. Leak of an anastomosis
     2. Leak of a suture line
     3. Stump insufficiency
     4. Other iatrogenic leaks

   C. Posttraumatic peritonitis
     1. Peritonitis after blunt abdominal trauma
     2. Peritonitis after penetrating abdominal trauma
     3. Other forms

III. **Tertiary peritonitis**
   A. Peritonitis without pathogens
   B. Peritonitis with fungi
   C. Peritonitis with low-grade pathogenic bacteria

IV. **Intra-abdominal abscess**
   A. Associated with primary peritonitis
   B. Associated with secondary peritonitis
   C. Associated with tertiary peritonitis

Phenomenological Classification

- Suppurative peritonitis
- Serofibrinous peritonitis
- Fibrinous-purulent peritonitis
- Fecal peritonitis
- Bilious peritonitis
- Hemorrhagic peritonitis
- Chemical peritonitis
- Talcum peritonitis
- Other forms

Classification According to the Spread of Infection

1. Diffuse peritonitis
2. Localized peritonitis
   - Intra-abdominal abscess
   - Interloop abscess
   - Douglas abscess
   - Subphrenic abscess
   - Subhepatic abscess
   - Retrocolic abscess
   - Pancreas abscess
   - Other abscesses

The accepted classification of intra-abdominal infection is subdivision into primary and secondary peritonitis, as shown below. This arcane classification has little clinical utility; clinicians referring to suppurative intra-abdominal infection use the term *peritonitis* without qualification. Some authors discuss tertiary peritonitis as a new entity seen in patients recovering from secondary peritonitis and experiencing an ongoing failure of host defenses without any further true infectious challenge.

Phenomenological Classification

This classification is based on the appearance of exudates. It is subdivided into serofibrinous (34.4% of all intra-abdominal inflammations) and fibrinous-purulent peritonitis (51.3%). It reflects the morphological substrate of various phases of inflammation. In addition, pathogenic factors are also considered, as reflected in the descriptions fecal (6.3%), biliary (5.2%), hemorrhagic (2.8%), chemical, and talcum peritonitis.

Classification by Spread of Infection

It is useful to classify peritonitis according to the extent of infection. Such a classification can help guide therapeutic strategies. Thus, we can distinguish cases of diffuse peritonitis that affect the whole abdominal cavity from localized cases of peritonitis or from intra-abdominal abscesses, for example, subphrenic, Douglas, or interloop abscesses.

Classification by Etiology

According to the route of infection, the disease has been grouped into primary and acute peritonitis.

I. Primary Peritonitis

Primary peritonitis refers to inflammation of the peritoneum from a suspected extraperitoneal source, often via hematogenous spread. It occurs as commonly in children as in adults, and more often in females than in males due to the open communication between the vagina and peritoneal cavity through the fallopian tubes. This extremely rare form of peritonitis is referred to as *hematogenous* peritonitis. In most cases it is caused by the hematogenous transport of bacteria or by the ascent of bacteria into the peritoneal cavity.

The pathogens normally seen are meningococci, pneumococci, gonococci, staphylococci, and hemolysing streptococci. In rare cases the infection is caused by anaerobic microorganisms or *Listeria monocytogenes*. Often the pathogens remain unidentified. The most important predisposing factor for primary peritonitis is cirrhosis of the liver. Juvenile peritonitis due to pneumococci is regarded as a typical form of primary peritonitis. The same goes for tuberculous peritonitis, which is often seen in underdeveloped countries.

A. Spontaneous peritonitis in children: The bacteria responsible for primary peritonitis are hemolytic streptococci and pneumococci. Two peaks of incidence are characteristic, one in the neonatal period and the other at ages four and five. The patients present with an acutely tender abdomen, fever, and leukocytosis. There may be a history of previous ear or upper respiratory infection. Children with nephrotic syndrome and systemic lupus erythematosus have a disproportionately high incidence. A Gram stain of a peritoneal tap may confirm the diagnosis. In the differential diagnosis, cystitis and pneumonia should be ruled out.

B. Spontaneous peritonitis in adults: Spontaneous peritonitis in adults is most commonly seen in patients with ascites due to cirrhosis. The spectrum of causative organisms has changed in the past decade; coliforms are now more frequent, and a distinction between primary and secondary peritonitis is now more difficult. Signs and symptoms do not differ greatly from those of acute peritonitis. The onset of symptoms may be slower.

C. Peritonitis with CAPD: Peritonitis is the dominating complication of continuous ambulatory peritoneal dialysis (CAPD) in patients with end-stage renal disease. The incidence varies from center to center. An overall average of 1.3 episodes per year has been estimated. Gram-positive microorganisms are the most frequent causes. *Pseudomonas aeruginosa* has been reported in 3.4% of the cases and generally cannot be cured by medical therapy only. Turbidity of the dialysate is the earliest sign and the only finding in one-fourth of the cases. If this is accompanied by abdominal pain or fever, prompt initiation of diagnostic laboratory studies and of therapy is required. Antibiotics have been administered intraperitoneally and intravenously, and a variety of regimens have been suggested. No single regimen has been shown to be the most efficacious in an appropriate clinical setup. Removal of the catheters is often required, and always necessary when the infection is due to *Pseudomonas aeruginosa*.

D. Tuberculous peritonitis: Tuberculous peritonitis, after a decrease in incidence during the past decade, is now becoming more common in Europe and North America with the increasing prevalence of AIDS due to HIV infection. It is still a serious primary problem in India, Southeast Asia, Africa, and Latin America. The tubercle bacillus presumably gains entry to the peritoneal cavity transmurally from diseased bowel, from tuberculous salpingitis, and from nephritis or other hematogenous distant sources. Clinically, most patients lack an obvious source; all patients, however, have such focus identified at autopsy. Patients usually have a positive tuberculin skin test. Two distinct clinical forms are manifested. The moist form consists of fever, ascites, abdominal pain, and weakness. The ascites is progressive and may become massive. The dry form presents without ascites. Diagnosis may be made most reliably by open or closed peritoneal biopsy. A peritoneal fluid tap will show mostly lymphocytes; acid-fast bacilli are rarely seen, and cultures are positive in less than half of all cases. Treatment is administration of antituberculous agents. Operations should be reserved for diagnosis, if needle biopsy fails, or for the treatment of such complications as fecal fistula.

II. Secondary or Perforation Peritonitis

This is the most common form of acute intra-abdominal infection. In major hospitals, about 80% of cases are due to a variety of primary necrotic lesions of the gastrointestinal tract and other intra-abdominal organs; 10 to 20% are seen in patients after abdominal operations (postoperative peritonitis).
In a series of 567 consecutive patients operated on for intra-abdominal infection over 7 years at General Hospital Hamburg-Altona, 14% occurred after a previous operation (table, p. 21). In 58% of patients, frank perforation of the GI tract due to peptic ulcer disease, diverticula, appendicitis, or a malignant lesion led to the infection. Bowel wall necrosis, either after strangulation due to incarcerated hernia or because of directly impaired vascular flow, was the cause of infection in 20% of the cases.

Peritonitis after perforation of stomach and duodenum: Infection after peptic ulcer perforation presents acutely; the patient is commonly able to give the exact time at which the perforation occurred. This form of peritonitis is chemical in nature initially, but with the passage of a short time becomes infected. The patient, however, most often seeks help very early due to the severe pain, and operative repair is often possible before systemic dissemination and organ failure have occurred. The proper management is simple closure. Some authors recommend additional definitive treatment of the peptic ulcer disease if the perforation is less than 12 hours old.
The high mortality of anastomotic leakage or suture-line breakdown after duodenal operations is explained by the fact that the duodenum is retroperitoneally fixed and cannot be exteriorized, and the source of infection often cannot be adequately controlled or closed. Consequently, infective material and proteolytic enzymes are continuously delivered into the peritoneal cavity, sustaining the infection.

Intra-abdominal infection after pancreatitis: Translocation of bacteria is probably the mechanism of progress from chemical inflammation to intra-abdominal infection. The combination of tissue necrosis due to proteolytic pancreatic juice and the presence of intestinal bacteria is the reason for the high mortality. The diagnosis of pancreatitis is not difficult; a history of midepigastric pain radiating to the right back in combination with an elevated amylase and lipase in serum and urine indicates the correct diagnosis. The transition from pancreatitis to diffuse peritonitis is more difficult to diagnose, and thus antimicrobial therapy is often started late when deterioration and multiple-organ system failure have occurred. In this type of advanced pathology, multiple planned reoperations *(Etappenlavage)* may be required.

Intra-abdominal infection after small bowel perforation: Symptoms of intra-abdominal infection after small bowel perforation fall into two major categories:
1. Ileus precedes peritonitis. The signs of bowel obstruction are the leading symptoms initially, gradually changing to symptoms of localized or diffuse peritonitis with fever and pathological white blood count findings.
2. Bowel wall necrosis is due to inadequate vascular supply or inflammation. Peritonitis may be diagnosed at a late stage due to the lack of initial symptoms. Often these patients are operated on very late in the evolution of their peritonitis, resulting in a mortality rate of more than 50%. This type of peritonitis is also seen after perforation of a typhoid small bowel lesion, a small bowel diverticulum, or other rare pathological entities.

Intra-abdominal infection and appendicitis: Formally speaking, appendicitis meets the criteria for local peritonitis, but, in most studies, it is not included under the term *secondary suppurative peritonitis* because of the localized inflammation and the extremely low mortality. If the appendix has perforated, however, it may become a life-threatening disease, especially when the omentum is not able to localize the inflammation and diffuse suppurative peritonitis results. The symptoms of appendicitis are outlined on p. 13. When peritonitis develops, there is usually a sudden deterioration in the clinical status. Treatment is likely to be successful because removing the appendix controls the source of infection. This explains the mortality of 13% in the series shown.
Disseminated intra-abdominal infection from appendicitis is not seen as often today as in the first decades of this century. Then, vital statistics

showed that appendicitis was the major cause of peritonitis seen in hospitals. Since the lifespan of patients has increased, other organ origins of peritonitis are now seen more often, and diseases of the aged—cancer and diverticulitis, for example—are more frequently the cause of intra-abdominal infection.

Intra-abdominal infection after colon perforation: Colon perforation due to diverticulitis or cancer is a common cause of diffuse, suppurative peritonitis. As shown in Chapter 4, a myriad of bacteria gain access to the peritoneal cavity through the perforated colon. This factor, together with the many associated diseases in the elderly patient population with colon disease, contributes to the high mortality. The basis for successful treatment, i.e., the elimination of the infectious source, is accomplished through colostomy or exterioration resection of the diseased colon. Another alternative for advanced stages is Etappenlavage, allowing for primary anastomosis.

Peritonitis after perforation of the genitourinary tract: A variety of conditions may cause peritonitis originating from the genitourinary tract. Ruptured perinephric abscess and chronic cystitis after radiation therapy for gynecological cancer are examples. Pelvic peritonitis due to sexually transmitted infection is seen in young women; there is usually acute, severe abdominal pain, and is easily diagnosed by Gram stain if suspected. Treatment with antimicrobials only is curative in nearly all cases. If tubo-ovarian abscess develops, operative treatment is required.

Postoperative peritonitis: Postoperative peritonitis is usually due to a leak from a suture line and is discovered only after delay—as a rule, between the fifth and seventh post-

operative days. Delay in diagnosis contributes to the high mortality. A suture-line leak is easier to repair if observed in the colon or small bowel, as compared to leaks of the upper GI tract. Upper GI tract pathology after an operation allows for only a limited therapeutic correction since these organs are fixed or closely attached to the retroperitoneum and the infectious source cannot be totally excluded or controlled under most circumstances. Resection of the anastomosis or of the diseased bowel segment is better than repair. Multiple planned relaparotomies (Etappenlavage) using a temporary abdominal closure device may be of particular benefit to this subset of intra-abdominal infections; at General Hospital Hamburg-Altona we were able to decrease the mortality to 23%.

Posttraumatic peritonitis: Peritonitis after blunt trauma may develop in patients with multiple injuries who have unrecognized additional intra-abdominal pathology, such as a ruptured mesenterium with obliteration of the vascular supply of the small or large bowel, or a frank bowel perforation. This type of intra-abdominal infection is usually severe because it is masked by other injuries. Treatment does not differ from that mentioned for intra-abdominal infection generally. Contamination of the abdominal cavity seen after penetrating abdominal trauma is usually not considered an intra-abdominal infection, although many trials testing the efficacy of antimicrobials erroneously use this subset of patients as representative of peritonitis.

III. Tertiary Peritonitis

Patients unable to contain an infection, whether because of inadequate host defense mechanisms or overwhelming infection, may go on to develop persistent diffuse peritonitis,

which Rotstein and Meakins have called tertiary peritonitis. The clinical picture is one of occult sepsis manifested by hyperdynamic cardiovascular parameters, low-grade fever, and a general hypermetabolic state. These patients have the clinical picture of sepsis without the presence of a well-defined focus of infection. They are subjected to numerous laparotomies to provide complete drainage of residual, infected fluid collections. These collections are different from true abscesses because they are not localized but tend to be diffuse. These patients frequently develop multiple-organ system failure and ultimately die. Bacteria of low pathogenic potential, usually selected by antimicrobial therapy, are isolated, including multi-resistant, coagulase-negative staphylococci, different species of pseudomonads, and fungi. These bacteria do not seem to be readily affected by antimicrobial treatment, suggesting a generalized failure of host defense.

Factors Influencing Mortality of IAI

Representative statistical information about IAI may be obtained by looking at patients managed operatively over a period of 9 years at General Hospital Hamburg-Altona. This hospital serves as the major medical facility in an urban area with a population of more than 400,000. Generally, all acute medical and surgical emergencies are

INTRA-ABDOMINAL INFECTIONS (n=567) AGE & MORTALITY

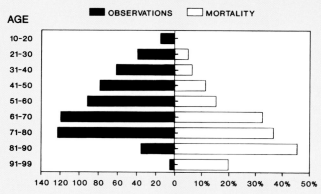

In recent years, more patients were referred from other, more distant hospitals, accounting for the increase in observations. Patients with acute appendicitis and acute cholecystitis were not included. Cases with perforated appendicitis were included only when advanced peritoneal inflammation was present. Patients with peritonitis after perforation of a peptic duodenal-gastric ulcer were generally included, which accounts for the relatively frequent observation of peritonitis

DURATION OF SYMPTOMS & MORTALITY

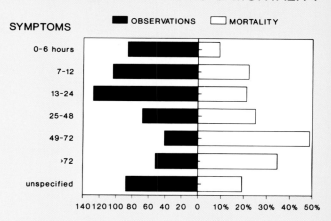

RISK FACTORS AT ADMISSION

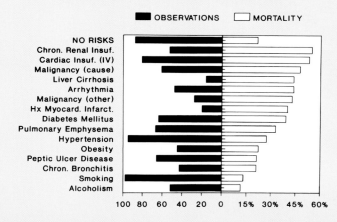

46

admitted to this hospital. A prehospital selection of patients, therefore, is unlikely to distort significantly the relative frequencies.

---

originating from the stomach and duodenum.

Detailed statistical analysis was performed on 567 patients from 1978 to 1984. During the last 2 years additional patients were referred from distant hospitals for Etappen-lavage treatment (see pp. 56–61). The higher number thus does not reflect an increase in the incidence of intra-abdominal infections. During 1981 the operating room was reconstructed and patients were not admitted for a period of 2 months.

WBC & MORTALITY

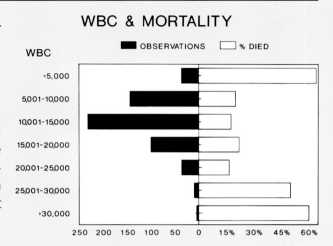

ETIOLOGY & MORTALITY

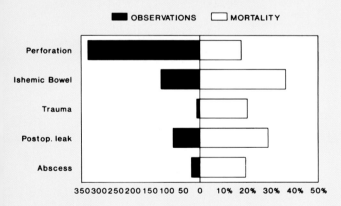

ANATOMICAL ORIGIN & MORTALITY

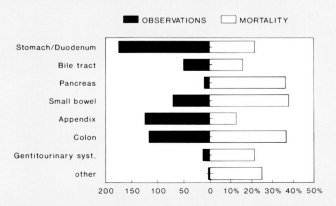

Peritonitis Index and Therapy: Scoring

To this day, the criteria for classification of peritonitis have failed to yield a reliable prognosis index, since the outcome of an abdominal inflammation depends on the complex interaction of numerous factors. Nevertheless, therapeutic progress requires that the disease be defined as exactly as possible and the patient's risks assessed precisely.

Prognosis indices should facilitate the comparison of treatment results from various clinics, which is necessary because the number of cases studied at an individual institution is seldom large enough to demonstrate significant differences between therapeutic modalities studied in controlled clinical studies.

To compare treatment results from different clinics using different therapy modalities, researchers have developed various scoring systems. All the systems aim at the quantification of risk relative to a certain form of peritonitis and patient risk factors influencing outcome. The compiled scores can then be used to facilitate comparisons between treatment results from different hospitals. Accordingly, patients with equal scores will have an equal mortality risk under standardized conditions. Such scoring systems help evaluate therapeutic strategies. If the results of a surgical or nonsurgical treatment yield a lower mortality than predicted by the score, the success of the chosen procedure is more likely to be as predicted than any historical comparison of treatment results might indicate.

The predictive indices used today have reached a remarkable degree of perfection. The most commonly used systems are the Mannheimer Peritonitis Index (MPI), the Peritonitis Index Altona (PIA II), and the Acute Physiology and Chronic Health Evaluation Score (APACHE II). While the first two systems base the prediction on anatomical and physiological findings, the latter accounts mainly for physiological changes. This score, therefore, can be used to assess therapeutic progress or deterioration whereas MPI and PIA are static and can be used only once, to determine the prognosis of an individual patient at the time of the initial operation. The limitation of all these systems is that about 10% of all patients cannot be classified correctly by any of the three.

Awaiting further results, the two Surgical Infections Societies propose that the APACHE II system be adopted for risk stratification of patients with intra-abdominal infections. This system has been validated in large independent patient populations and used in several studies of intra-abdominal infections. The APACHE II system has a large range of scores with small increments, each of which contributes to calculation of the risk, and the score value is translatable into a mortality risk level that compares favorably with the observed mortality. For this purpose, a weight factor of -0.273 for intra-abdominal infections has recently been determined in a multicenter trial of the Surgical Infection Society—Europe.

Finally, it should be noted that the scoring systems are designed not to establish a prognosis for an individual patient but to facilitate comparisons between larger patient populations receiving specific treatment. Based on such a comparison, we can then determine which treatment is superior.

The Mannheim Peritonitis Index (MPI)

This index was developed by Linder and Wacha. Its prognostic accuracy was validated by studies with large patient collectives. MPI is problematic in that it excludes intra-abdominal infections due to appendicitis, endoscopic perforation, pancreatitis, mesenteric infarction, and post-operative peritonitis. Hence it is unknown if MPI is applicable to all patients with intra-abdominal infections usually observed in studies to improve treatment modalities. For a score of up to 15, the expected mortality is virtually 0; up to 21, the risk of death is less than 6%. This score has recently been considerably improved and may be used as a reference.

The Peritonitis Index Altona (PIA)

The PIA system was developed at the Altona General Hospital. As with the MPI, the PIA system is based on anamnestically derived data, intra-operative findings, and physiologic information. PIA II, the refined version of the original index, yields a more precise definition of the patient population.

In the development of PIA II, all 567 patients operated for intra-abdominal infections between 1978 and 1984 were included. The definition of intra-abdominal infection did not include cholecystitis and appendicitis without perforation. First, the variables recorded were evaluated with respect to their influence on the target variable—survivor or non-survivor—utilizing the Yates corrected chi-square test. For this purpose qualitative variables were transformed into quantitative data.

Since the aim was to develop an index describing the prognosis of patients before any specific therapy was initiated, only information available pre- and intra-operatively was used. During the selection of criteria, only those risk factors that were sufficiently frequent, clearly defined, simply evaluated, and reproducible were utilized. Therefore the list obtained from chronic health evaluation was considerably reduced. Insulin-dependent diabetes mellitus, a well-defined variable, proved to be an important risk factor. It was not possible, however, to omit the highly predictive variable of congestive heart failure, although a range of definitions was used. Also, aspects of etiology and origin of infection as well-defined variables as assessed at the primary operation

were utilized. Only two laboratory findings (leucocyte count and serum creatinine) were accepted by discriminant analysis. They could be affected only moderately by initial therapy.

The patient population was then randomly assigned to a test group (60% of all patients) or to a validation group (40% of all patients). In the test group cross-tabulation with the outcome of peritonitis was performed for combinations of variables including disease origin and etiology, and the relative mortality was noted. Those groups with mortality risk most deviant from the average were listed and subjected to multivariate discriminant analysis. With this method the index for an individual patient was calculated according to:

$$C = c(1)V(1) + c(2)V(2) + \ldots + c(n)V(n) + K$$

where C = Index, $c(1)\ldots c(n)$ = coefficients (weighting factors), V = value of the variable, and K = constant.

The last step was to validate the score calculated on the remaining 40% of patients not used to calculate the score.

Stepwise discriminant analysis ranked the entrance variables according to their power in discriminating between the target variables and attributing a discrimination factor to each. These factors were transformed to ease clinical applicability into a score with zero as a midpoint. Negative values predicted an increased likelihood of death; positive values, an increased probability of survival. The confidence limits were 97.5% correct prediction at scores below -1.315 and above $+1.315$, and 68.5% at scores below -0.275 and above $+0.275$, respectively. In the patients studied the scores ranged between -7.6 and 2.7.

The PIA II score classified 89% of all test group patients correctly. The validation of the score in the unknown patient group correctly classified 81.4% of cases. Additionally, an equation was developed to calculate an individual's mortality risk from the score:

$$Px = \frac{e^{2.8(PIAx)}}{1 + e^{2.8(PIAx)}}$$

where Px = probability for death or survival and $PIAx$ = individual score of patient x. The mean of all Px's of a patient population may then be used to evaluate results of a new treatment modality.

Calculation of Probability of Death

The risk of hospital death predicted for a given patient population is assessed by calculating the mean of R of all patients or appropriate subgroups. R is the risk of hospital death of a single patient.

To calculate R for a single patient with acute suppurative peritonitis, use the following equation:.

R = Risk of hospital death

$$R = \frac{EXP(AW)}{EXP(1 + AW)}$$

since

$$A = \ln \frac{R}{1 - R}$$

AW = (APACHE II score $\times$ 0.146) + W

where

W = W1 + W2 + W3 = -3.15

since

W1 = -3.517 (Unspecific weight)

W2 = $+0.603$ (Weight for post-emergency surgery)

W3 = -0.273 (Diagnostic category weight for intra-abdominal infections)

Hence:

$$R = \frac{EXP((APACHE\ II \times 0.146) - 3.15)}{1 + (EXP((APACHE\ II \times 0.146) - 3.15))}$$

where EXP(n) gives e (2.7182818 . . .) to the exponent of n.

Bibliography

Knaus WA, et al. Crit Care Med 13:818–829, 1985.

Wittmann DH, Nyström P-O. Surg Res Commun 8:27, 1990.

APACHE II Score and IAI: Practical Application

Make copies of these pages and use one set for each patient.

Patient's name: _____
Date of Birth: _____ [1] Age: _____ Hospital _____
[2] Sex: _____ [3] Race: _____
[4] Duration of initial, pertinent symptoms: Days: _____ Hours: _____
[5] Admission to ICU from Operating Room .... [yes] [no] Floor .... [yes] [no]
Other Hospital ....[yes] [no]
[6] Diagnosis: _____
[7] Operation: _____
[8] Intra-operative complications: _____
[9] Time from hospital admission to ICU admission: Days: _____ Hours: _____

APACHE II Assessment Sheet

	POINTS	+4	+3	+2	+1	0	+1	+2	+3	+4
TEMPERATURE -- rectal Centigrade: (°C = (°F - 32) x 5/9)	( )	<30	30-31.9	32-33.9	34-35.9	36-38.4	38.5-38.9		39-40.9	≥41
MEAN BLOOD PRESSURE -- mm Hg (2 x diastolic BP + systolic BP)/3	( )	<50		50-69		70-109		110-129	130-159	≥160
HEART RATE (ventricular response)	( )	<40	40-54	55-69		70-109		110-139	140-179	≥180
RESPIRATORY RATE -- total (nonventilated or ventilated rate)	( )	<6		6-9	10-11	12-24	25-34		35-49	≥50
HEMATOCRIT (%)	( )	<20		20.0-29.9		30.0-45.9	46.0-49.9	50.0-59.9		≥60
WHITE BLOOD COUNT (total, mm³) (in 1,000's)	( )	<1		1-2.9		3-14.9	15-19.9	20-39.9		≥40
ARTERIAL pH (arterial blood gases, ABGs)	( )	<7.15	7.15-7.24	7.25-7.32		7.33-7.49	7.5-7.59		7.6-7.69	≥7.7
SERUM SODIUM (mg/dL)	( )	<111	111-119	120-129		130-149	150-154	155-159	160-179	≥180
SERUM POTASSIUM (mg/dL)	( )	<2.5		2.5-2.9	3.0-3.4	3.5-5.4	5.5-5.9		6.0-6.9	≥7
SERUM CREATININE (mg/dL) Double the creatinine point score for acute renal failure (ARF) ○	( )			<0.6		0.6-1.4		1.5-1.9	2.0-3.4	≥3.5
SERUM CO₂ (venous mg/dL) [NOT PREFERRED. Use only if no ABGs available; substitutes for pH and assumes normal oxygenation]	( )		15-17.9	18-21.9		22-31.9	32-40.9		41-51.9	≥52
OXYGENATION: A - aDO₂ or PaO₂ (mm Hg) if FiO₂ ≥ 50, then record A - aDO₂, A - aDO₂ = [FiO₂ (713) - PaCO₂ - PaO₂]; if FiO₂ < 50, then record only PaO₂.	( )	<55	55-60		61-70	≥70 / <200		200-349	350-499	≥500

Neurologic Points for GLASGOW COMA SCORE (GCS):
To calculate: Neurologic Points = (15-actual GCS);

Neurologic Points:	15 - _____ = _____ ; (CGS)	Neurologic Points: ( )

A. Total ACUTE PHYSIOLOGY SCORE (APS): Sum of the 12 individual variable points ( )

PROBABILITY OF DEATH _____ %

Sum of: A _____ + B _____ + C _____ = _____ A APS points B Age points C Chronic Health Points

Age points: 0 1 2 3 4 5 6 7 8 9 10 11 12 *Use specific weight

Chronic Health Points _____

Total APACHE II ( )

50

APACHE II Score

The APACHE II score is calculated by adding Acute Physiology Score (APS) points, Age points and Chronic Health Evaluation (CHE) points

$$\text{APACHE II} = \text{Sum of } [A]+[B]+[C]$$

[A] APS points: [____] enter fom section   [A]

[B] Age points: [____] enter from section   [B]

[C] Chronic health points: [____] enter from section   [C]

Total APACHE II points: .. [_____] Sum of [A]+[B]+[C]

to calculate Predicted Mortality use formula of page 50

$$R = \frac{\text{Exp}((\text{APACHE} \times 0.146) - 3.15)}{1 + (\text{Exp}((\text{APACHE} \times 0.146) - 3.15))}$$

$$\begin{aligned} AW &= (\text{Apache-II} \times 0.146) - W \\ &= ([\quad] \times 0.146) - 3.15 \\ &= [\quad] \end{aligned}$$

> Enter APACHE II and calculate AW

$$R = \text{EXP} (AW / 1 + AW)$$

$$R = \text{EXP} (\underline{\quad\quad\quad\quad}) = [\quad\quad]\%$$

PERCENT PREDICTED MORTALITY

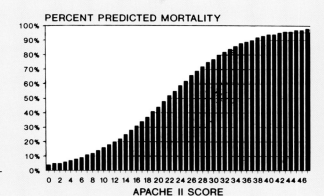

Weight for IAI -0.273

APACHE-II score and predicted mortality for intra-abdominal infections.

SECTION [C]

Chronic Health Evaluation (CHE)

If the patient's past medical history indicates a serious pre-morbidity in any of the 5 categories listed, assign (+ 5) Chronic Health Points
1. Liver .... [yes]/[no]
2. Cardiovascular .... [yes]/[no]
4. Renal function .... [yes]/[no]
3. Respiratory: .... [yes]/[no]
5. Immuno-compromised: .... [yes]/[no]

If any of the 5 CHE categories is answered with [yes] give +5 points

CHRONIC HEALTH POINTS (CHE) .... [____] = [C]

Definitions
Organ insufficiency or immuno-compromised state must have been evident prior to this hospital admission and conform to the following criteria:

1. Liver: Biopsy proven cirrhosis and documented portal hypertension; episodes of past upper GI bleeding attributed to portal hypertension; prior episodes of hepatic failure/encephalopathy/coma.

2. Cardiovascular: New York Heart Association Class IV heart failure.

3. Respiratory: Chronic restrictive, obstructive, or vascular disease resulting in severe exercise restriction, e.g.: unable to climb stairs or perform household duties; chronic hypoxia, hypercapnia, polycythemia, pulmonary hypertension (> 40 mmHg); respirator dependency.

4. Renal: Patients receiving chronic dialysis.

5. Immuno-compromised: The patient has received therapy that suppresses resistance to infection,
e.g.   immuno-suppression, chemotherapy, radiation, long-term steroids or recent high dose steroids, has a disease that is sufficiently advanced to suppress resistance to infection,
e.g: - leukemia,   - lymphoma, - AIDS.

SECTION [A]
Acute Physiology Score (APS)

The Acute Physiology Score is the sum of 12 physiologic points including Neurologic Points (15-Glasgow Coma Score)

Assessment of Glasgow Coma Score

A) EYES ARE OPENED:

B) MOTOR - Response	
after verbal stimuli	(+6)
after pain stimuli	(+5)
uncontrolled movements	(+4)
spontaneously	(+4)

sponataneously	(+4)	flexion reflexes	(+4)
when spoken to	(+3)	decortication rigidity	(+3)
when in pain	(+2)	decerebration rigidity	(+2)
no response	(+1)	no response	(+1)

C) STATE OF CONSCIOUSNESS

For spontaneously breathing patients:		**For intubated patients**	
oriented, converses	(+5)	oriented,could converse	(+5)
disoriented, can converse	(+4)		
answers are confused	(+3)	conversing questionable	(+3)
answers incomprehensible	(+2)		
patient unresponsive	(+1)	generally unresponsive	(+1)

ACUTE PHYSIOLOGY SCORE: .... [_____]=[A]

SECTION [B]
AGE POINTS: Assign points to age as follows:

Age (years)	<44	45-54	55-64	65-74	>75
Points	0	2	3	5	6

AGE POINTS: .... [_____]=[B]

The therapy of intra-abdominal infections is based on three principles:
- Elimination of noxae by surgical procedures
- Calculated antibiotic therapy
- Intensive-care treatment for the control of secondary and tertiary damage

Surgical Sanitation of the Focus

This is the most important prerequisite for the successful therapy of intra-abdominal infections. The operation should be performed as early as possible in order to prevent further influx of toxic material into the peritoneal cavity. Additionally, surgical therapy is designed to eliminate pus and massive bacterial invasion.

Antimicrobial Chemotherapy

This is directed against the specific pathogens at the origin of infection. It should *not* be begun before the bacterial inoculum has been reduced by the initial operation, to reduce endotoxin deluge and to allow for confirmation of the diagnosis and proper pathogen identification by sampling pus from the abdominal cavity.

Critical or Intensive-Care Treatment

Critical care should begin immediately after the first examination. Initially, it is designed to repair prior damage so as to reduce the operative risk. It should, however, never delay the operation substantially.

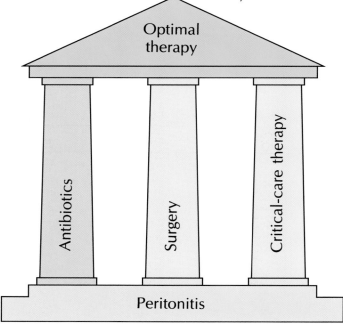

Optimal therapy

Antibiotics — Surgery — Critical-care therapy

Peritonitis

The operative management of peritonitis eliminates the cause of the disease and cleans the abdominal cavity, thus reducing the bacterial challenge.

Calculated antibacterial chemotherapy kills pathogens beyond the reach of surgical measures.

Critical-care therapy enables proper surgical management of the disease, repairs secondary organ damage, and controls overwhelming pathophysiological reactions of the organism.

The goal of therapy is to interrupt the pathophysiological processes causing intra-abdominal infections by:
1. Eliminating the source of infection
2. Controlling subsequent damage

Three Objectives

1. The elimination of the source of infection by adequate elimination of the focus of infection and safe control of these measures.

2. The elimination of toxic material by adequate surgical cleaning of the abdominal cavity—if necessary, in a stepwise procedure—and by calculated antimicrobial therapy directed against causative agents.

3. The control of systemic damages by intensive-care therapy that manages and reverses pathophysiological consequences of peritonitis.

The Interplay of Therapeutic Measures

The surgical elimination of the infectious focus is the most important prerequisite for successful therapy of intra-abdominal infections. An adequate elimination of the source of infection is the only guarantee against a further influx of bacteria-carrying, infective-toxic material into the abdominal cavity and thus against further damage to the entire organism. For this reason, surgical therapy has top priority.

So as not to delay the surgical management of the cause of peritonitis, we must make sure that:
1. Antibiotic therapy does not begin before the operation and the surgical reduction of the bacterial count. Otherwise, the rapid destruction of bacteria in the presence of potent antibiotics can result in overwhelming endotoxemia. This can precipitate a breakdown of circulatory regulation before surgery, making the patient temporarily inoperable, and delay operative management.

2. Critical-care treatment prepares the patient for surgery, so that the focus of infection can be sanitized as fast as possible.
3. Diagnostic procedures are restricted to those absolutely necessary for determining the cause of peritonitis. Invasive devices can be inserted during the operation.

Any postponement of surgical intervention may lead to additional damage to the total organism and increases the risk of multiple-organ failure.

53

Operative Therapy

Operative therapy encompasses the surgical management of infectious foci and the cleaning of the abdominal cavity, eliminating purulent necrotic material. Traditionally accomplished in one single procedure, this has become the standard operative management of peritonitis.

Introduction

Intra-abdominal infections are treated according to principles established during the first two decades of this century. These include one operative procedure, antibacterial treatment with drugs, and support of functional impairment. The operation is considered to be the most important step. Its purpose is to evacuate purulent necrotic material from the abdominal cavity and to eliminate the infectious source. This therapeutic strategy has become the standard operative management of intra-abdominal infections. Overall mortality was reduced from 90% at the turn of the century to about 40% in 1926 (p. 8). Further improvements were expected to follow the introduction of more potent antimicrobials and better intensive-care facilities. The mortality rates, however, remained unchanged. Consequently, during the past decade, surgeons have explored new operative approaches to improve the ultimate outcome. Three basically different methods have emerged:

1. Postoperative lavage procedures
2. Open management of the abdomen
3. Planned multiple reoperations (Etappenlavage)

While the different postoperative lavage procedures were designed to treat all forms and stages of IAI, the open management and the stepwise repair procedures were developed to treat patients at high risk with diffuse advanced purulent peritonitis only. Patients qualifying for the latter two procedures usually have a predicted mortality exceeding 50%.

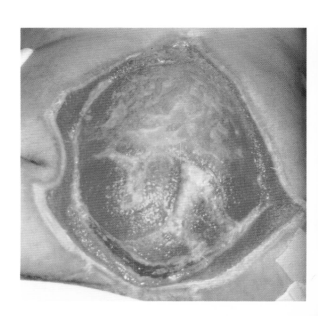

Late stage of the open abdomen technique. There is fresh granulation tissue covering abdominal organs. The opening corresponds to the size of the resulting incisional hernia.

With the availability of improved diagnostic methods such as sonography and computed tomography, the incision into the abdomen has become more precise and directed to the focus of the disease. Only in rare cases is the abdomen opened without knowledge of the source of infection.

1. Incision

With the availability of improved diagnostic methods such as sonography and computed tomography, the incision into the abdomen has become more precise and directed to the focus of the disease. Only in rare cases is the abdomen opened without knowledge of the source of infection. Consequently, the surgeon can dismiss the concept of midline laparotomy in favor of a more physiological transverse laparotomy. This incision allows an adequate inspection of the abdominal organs and is much better tolerated by these patients. Moreover, the contraction of musculature along the median line leading to wound dehiscence is avoided. Transverse incisions have also been shown to have a better healing tendency. Pararectal and other incisions have become obsolete. They cannot be extended when pathological findings of the abdomen are greater than expected. In any case, the incision must be large enough to allow optimal elimination of the focus.

2. Sanitation of Foci

The complete removal of origin of infection is a prerequisite for therapeutic success. The strategic importance of this effort in the overall concept of peritonitis therapy can hardly be overestimated. The elimination of the infectious source or focus in conjunction with the cleansing of the abdominal cavity reduces the infectious inoculum to a size treatable by antibiotic therapy. Even intensive-care efforts cannot control toxic organ damage without focal sanitation, as the infectious material will continue to flow into the peritoneal cavity and eventually reach the circulatory system.

When the infectious focus cannot be sanitized adequately, the prognosis is poor. For example, in the upper gastrointestinal tract, proper sanitation sometimes is virtually impossible, since these organs are retroperitoneally fixed. The mortality rate of this type of infection is much higher than in lower gastrointestinal tract peritonitis, where exteriorization of the focus as an ultimate step is always possible. Therefore, surgical efforts must be complete and adequate. If complete focal removal cannot be realized in one operation, multiple operations should be planned.

The frequently stated objection that the least invasive measure in this situation is also the best is not only false; it is also dangerous. The assumed safety is, in fact, an illusion.

3. Cleaning the Abdominal Cavity

There are various approaches to cleaning the abdominal cavity. First, there is simple cleaning by swabbing the cavity. Next, there is extensive intraoperative lavage with up to about 10 L of saline or Ringer's lactate. Then there is the continuous postoperative lavage using drains. Finally, there is the method of radical debridement.

Debridement

Debridement of dead tissue and elimination of bacteria and toxins may be accomplished by the various techniques listed below.

3.1 Swabbing

Debates continue to rage on whether it is better to wash or to swab out toxic material from the abdominal cavity. The advocates of pure swabbing argue that the import of additional fluid into the abdominal cavity shields bacteria from macrophage phagocytosis. Indeed, only a few clinics prefer swabbing as the only method today. Controlled studies on this question have not been reported. Based on case reports, the therapeutic success of swabbing does not seem to differ essentially from other methods.

3.2 Intraoperative Lavage

This term is used for the extensive intraoperative lavage of the entire abdominal cavity. The surgeon administers 0.5 to 1 L of physiological saline or Ringer's solution into the abdominal cavity, washes out pus, feces, and necroses, and then aspirates the fluid. This procedure is repeated until the suctioned fluid runs clear. Usually, this requires a total administration of 8 to 12 L. Sometimes antimicrobial substances are added to the lavage fluid. The efficacy of this measure alone, however, has not been persuasively shown in controlled studies. Polyvinylpyrrolidone-iodine (PVP-I) should not be added to peritoneal lavage fluid. In animal experiments, the use of PVP-I has led to the death of the animals, whereas saline-lavaged animals survived. Iodine is highly toxic for cells in the peritoneum. The FDAs of most countries do not allow the use of PVP iodine for intraperitoneal application.

3.3 Continuous Lavage

For a number of years, various authors have promoted the continuous posterior-to-anterior lavage of the abdominal cavity. In this method, the abdominal wounds are not completely closed; instead they are covered by drains, for example. Infusion of irrigation fluid into the posterior region of the abdominal cavity is supposed to wash out debris, toxins, and bacteria anteriorly out of the abdominal wound.

A number of authors support a continuous postoperative lavage. In this method, four to six Tenckhoff catheters are placed in the abdominal cavity and lavage fluid is infused for an hour, and then the process is reversed. Controlled studies comparing continuous lavage to the standard therapy have had differing results. In most studies, the number of cases examined do not justify significant conclusions as to one method's superiority. Often drains occlude. There is no way to ensure that all diseased areas of the abdominal cavity are washed. Drains also may erode and perforate intestines, contributing to new complications.

3.4 Open Abdomen

In this method, which in recent years has been used mainly by French surgeons, the abdominal cavity is left open following laparotomy. The treatment concept appears to be the logical continuance of surgical principles to incise and evacuate a surgical infection through the open wound *(ubi pus, ibi evacua).* An important advantage of this method is that it counteracts deleterious rising of intra-abdominal pressure induced by inflammation and edema of the peritoneum. Forceful closing as seen in the standard management induces basal atelectasis formation with subsequent pneumonia, and impairs hemodynamic and renal function. Problems with the open-abdomen method lie in the frequent occurrence of intestinal fistulae. Intestines perforate if augmented intraluminal pressure is not counteracted. Also, definitive closure of the abdominal wall is impossible, and huge incisional hernias require secondary repair. Some surgeons combine the open-abdomen method with continuous postoperative abdominal lavage, a method that is similar to the dorsoventral lavage method mentioned earlier *(see photo).*

4. Critique of "Abdominal Toilet" Methods

All cleaning methods have disadvantages. With pure swabbing there is the danger that the peritoneal cavity is not sufficiently cleaned. The bacterial inoculum as well as the remaining necrotic material can override the phagocytic capacity of the organism. In the forms of lavage, bacteria are suspended in liquid and thereby removed from host defenses. In the continuous lavage methods, pathways for the liquid sooner or later develop and, ultimately, only small areas of the abdominal cavity are actually washed. In addition, drainage tracts are apt to clog, leading to erosion and intestinal perforation. Formation of intestinal fistulae is another serious complication. Consequently, the open-abdomen method has lost its popularity.

Etappenlavage combines the advantages of the open abdomen technique with closure of the abdominal wall, by utilizing a device for temporary abdominal closure (TAC). The most useful device for TAC is the artificial burr. It enables gradual approximation of the fascias, along with the decrease of the abdominal edema, and replacement by a smaller device is no longer necessary.

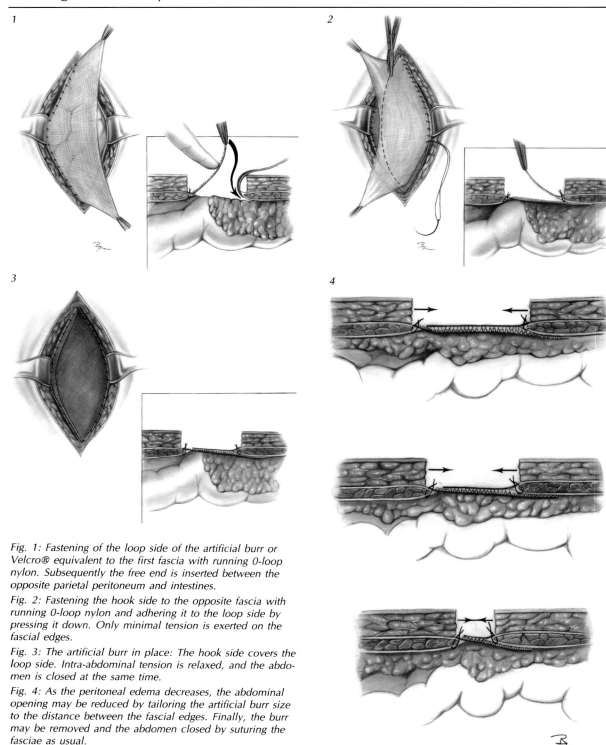

Fig. 1: Fastening of the loop side of the artificial burr or Velcro® equivalent to the first fascia with running 0-loop nylon. Subsequently the free end is inserted between the opposite parietal peritoneum and intestines.

Fig. 2: Fastening the hook side to the opposite fascia with running 0-loop nylon and adhering it to the loop side by pressing it down. Only minimal tension is exerted on the fascial edges.

Fig. 3: The artificial burr in place: The hook side covers the loop side. Intra-abdominal tension is relaxed, and the abdomen is closed at the same time.

Fig. 4: As the peritoneal edema decreases, the abdominal opening may be reduced by tailoring the artificial burr size to the distance between the fascial edges. Finally, the burr may be removed and the abdomen closed by suturing the fasciae as usual.

New Methods of Operative Management

Operating adequately in extremely advanced stages of peritonitis is fraught with technical limitations. 15% of all patients present with such an advanced stage of peritonitis. The limitations of standard operative management have been one reason for a stagnating mortality of peritonitis following standardization of operative technique by Kirschner in 1926. Clearly, the continuously high mortality of peritonitis

Etappenlavage

Etappenlavage (ETL) combines the advantages of the open-abdomen technique with the closure of the abdominal wall, thus preventing a buildup of intra-abdominal pressure, without the risk of intestinal fistula formation. It represents a commitment to re-explore the patient's abdomen at regular intervals after the original corrective operation. This ensures gentle elimination of the infected source and promotes maximal reduction of toxic necrotic material by daily abdominal cleansing. Intra-abdominal complications are promptly recognized, and immediate repair effected. Like the technique of leaving the abdomen open, it takes into account the increased intra-abdominal pressure, but unlike the open-abdomen technique it is rarely complicated by intestinal fistulae. The abdominal cavity is not closed by suturing the fascia. Instead, different devices for temporary abdominal closure are used to cover the abdominal aperture, allowing for sufficient space within the abdominal cavity to contain the inflamed and edematous intra-abdominal organs. In addition, primary intra-abdominal anastomoses can be sutured. Deviation colostomies are less frequently required and no longer prolong patients' suffering. Necroses occurring in the course of the infection on anastomoses or sutures, especially on retroperitoneally fixed upper abdominal organs, can be recognized at an early stage and treated accordingly. This therapeutic concept is extraordinarily flexible, allowing for strategic adaptation during the progression of the disease. In comparison, the rigid concept of a single "final" operation forfeits immediate reactions to pathological processes.

Etappenlavage for Diffuse Peritonitis: Development of an Operative Technique

Author	Device used for temporary abdominal closure	Interval between relaparotomies (hr)	Died/total	Mortality (%)
Hay et al. (1979)	Marlex® mesh	24	9/26	35
Fagniez et al. (1979)	Polyurethane foam	Variable	21/70	30
Goris (1980)	Marlex® mesh	Variable	13/26	50
Kerremans and Penninckx (1982)	Retention sutures	48	15/39	38
Teichmann et al. (1982)	Retention sutures	24	4/21	19
Wouters et al. (1983)	Marlex® mesh	Variable	4/20	20
Penninckx et al. (1983)	Retention sutures	48	9/31	29
Stone et al. (1984)	Zipper	Variable	7/36	19
Bartels et al. (1985)	Retention sutures	48	14/46	30
Muhrer et al. (1985)	Vicryl® mesh	48	11/27	41
Heddrich et al. (1986)	Marlex® + zipper	48	2/10	20
Teichmann et al. (1986)	Slide fastener	24	14/61	23
Garcia-Sabrido et al. (1988)	Zipper-mesh	24	15/64	23
Wittman (1990)	Artificial burr	24	28/117	24

Source: World Journal of Surgery 14(2):146, 1990.

during subsequent decades was unacceptable. Descriptions of new methods were published in the early 1980s and were thought to establish a therapeutic concept of more effective operative treatment. Advances in critical-care treatment based on better understanding of the pathophysiology form the foundation for a radical approach of multiple planned laparotomies, called Etappenlavage.

Indication for Etappenlavage (Planned Relaparotomy)

1. Mortality prediction <50% (APACHE-II >21) and/or poor patient condition precluding definitive repair
2. Source of infection not eliminated
3. Necrosectomy uncomplete
4. Bowel ischemia
5. Multiple previous procedures
6. Excessive peritoneal edema
7. Uncontrollable hemorrhage → packing

Operative Technique

First Operation

Upon the decision to perform multiple operations, made at the time of the original corrective operation, the artificial burr may be sutured to the fascial edges of the longitudinal or transverse abdominal incision. The two sheets of the artificial burr are first trimmed to the size of the incision by cutting off the edges with a pair of scissors. Then the loop or velours sheet is sutured to the first fascial edge with a 0-loop nylon running suture. The loops face outwards; the slightly enforced back of the loop side covers the omentum over the bowel. Once the loop sheet is fastened to the fascia, its free part is gently slipped underneath the opposing fascia (Fig. 1, p. 57).

Then the hook side is sutured to the second fascia, again using 0-loop nylon in a simple continuous running technique (Fig. 2, p. 57). The closure is terminated by simply pressing the hook side gently upon the loop side while exerting a slight tension via the hook sheet on the attached fascia. This will prevent the fascias from retraction and ease reapproximation once the increased intra-abdominal pressure has subsided. The abdominal aperture, however, is left wide enough to avoid any tension or increased intra-abdominal pressure.

Relaparotomy

Relaparotomy is easily performed by shearing the hook sheet off the loop sheet. This is preferably done in the operating room, but may also be performed in the ICU for, for example, rapid diagnosis of acute deteriorations due to dead bowel. Both sheets are then extroverted and pulled over the wound edges. The abdomen can then be explored in the usual way. The artificial burr does not interfere with surgical manipulations. Upon termination of the operation, the two sheets of artificial burrs are approximated in the same fashion as at the first operation. Usually, at subsequent operations, the abdominal aperture may be decreased in size by pulling the fascial edge via the sheet of the artificial burr.

At the last operation, which may be the tenth planned relaparotomy, the suture is removed, thus detaching the artificial burr sheets from the fascia. The abdomen may then be closed by suturing the two fascial borders in a typical way.

Advantages of Etappenlavage	Advantages That Must Be Noted in Relation to the Disadvantages of a Standard Therapy
• Effective elimination of the cause	
• Effective reduction of bacterial inoculum	• Uncertain elimination of the cause
• Effective elimination of toxins	• Insufficient reduction of bacterial counts
• No drainage complications	• Insufficient elimination of toxins
• Flexible therapeutic concept	• Possible drainage complications
• Timely diagnosis and therapy of complications	• Rigid therapeutic concept
	• Delayed reinterventions due to dependency on indirect parameters of GI tract leaks

The Concept of Etappenlavage

Etappenlavage (ETL) combines the advantages of the open-abdomen technique with the closure of the abdominal wall, thus preventing a buildup of intra-abdominal pressure and avoiding the risk of intestinal fistula formation. It represents a commitment made to re-explore the patient's abdomen at regular intervals after the original corrective operation. This ensures gentle elimination of the infected source and promotes maximal repair and reduction of toxic necrotic material by daily abdominal cleansing.

Chronological Sequence of Scheduled Reintervention ETL

Fig. 1: Sanitation of focus. Feculent pus within the abdominal cavity stemming from a small bowel perforation needs to be removed as soon as this material has been cultured aerobically and anaerobically. Upon completion of the lavage, few bacteria are left and antimicrobial therapy may be started without too high a risk for overwhelming endotoxinemia.

Fig. 2: Cleansing of the abdominal cavity. This is best done by lavage with 8–10 L of Ringer's solution. No fluid is left within the abdomen, and macrophage activity should not be impaired.

Fig. 3: Elimination of the infectious source. The next step is to make sure that the source of infection is closed or exteriorized to prevent further delivery of bacteria, toxins, and necroses into the abdomen.

Fig. 4: Suturing anastomoses. Anastomoses may be repaired primarily, since their healing can be monitored during subsequent Etappenlavages. Anastomoses done with a stapler are usually safer since their prefixed distance is based on normal rather than inflamed and edematous bowel. Bowel anastomoses sutured in initial stages of peritonitis may leak, because the sutures become loose as the inflammatory edema decreases.

Fig. 5: Suturing the artificial burr to the fascia. Temporary abdominal closure is best accomplished by suturing each sheet of the artificial burr to the opposing fascia. Here the fuzz side is already in place, and the hook side is fastened to the fascia by running 0-loop nylon.

Fig. 6: Tension-free adaptation closure, no drainage. The artificial burr closed. Note the large gap between the wound edges well accommodating intra-abdominal organs without undue pressure. The abdomen is relaxed, and impairment of renal, pulmonary, and hemodynamic function is avoided.

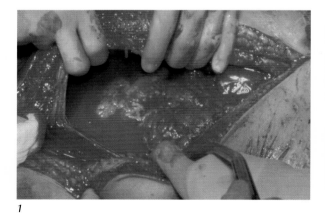

1

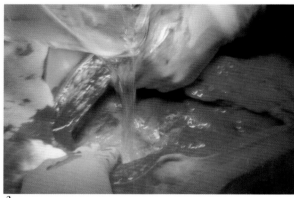

2

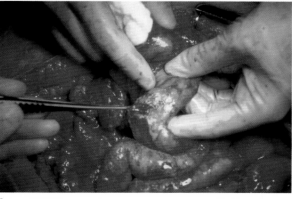

3

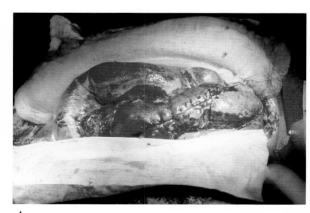

4

60

Etappenlavage is characterized by:
- Sanitation of focus
- Adaptation closure, no drainage
- Reintervention every 24 hours, lavage
- Closure of abdominal wall when exudate is clear, no drainage

Relaparotomies Are Performed Every 24 Hours

Fig. 7: Sequel operation after 24 hours, control of focus. The artificial burr is opened easily by pulling the hook side (peeling off).

Fig. 8: Inspection and lavage of abdominal cavity. Further necroses may be removed and anastomoses inspected.

Fig. 9: Inspection of anastomosis; anastomotic healing.

Fig. 10: Reopening of abdomen. As peritoneal edema decreases, the artificial burr may be trimmed by cutting the borders. The fascial edges may be approximated more closely as shown here. Finally, the artificial burr is removed and the abdomen may be closed in the regular way by suturing the fascial edges.

Final Operation

The abdomen may be definitively closed without drainage when most of the necroses are eliminated, the source of infection is secured, the APACHE II predicts an improved prognosis, the exudate becomes clear, and good intestinal motility is seen.

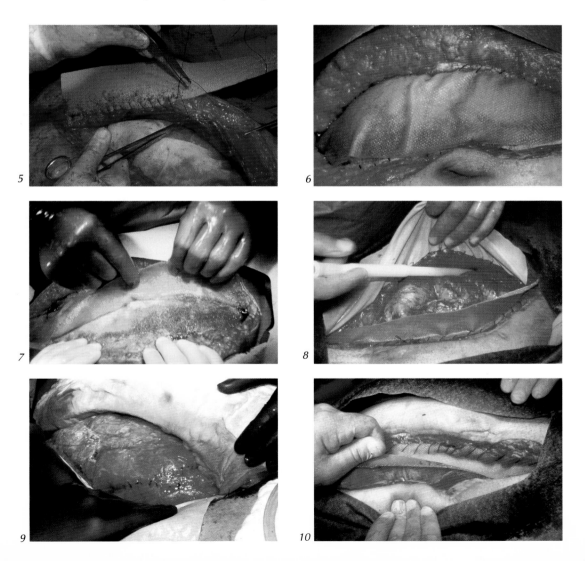

5

6

7

8

9

10

To facilitate temporary abdominal closure (TAC) and reopening of the abdomen, several ingeneous techniques have been promoted. Retention wires were used first. Then a zipper, first employed in surgery in 1936 by Strauss, was successfully sutured to the fascial edges for temporary abdominal closure. Later, when the negative influence of increased abdominal pressure on pulmonary, cardiac, and renal function became apparent, retention sutures or simple zippers for TAC were re-

Methods for Temporary Abdominal Closure (TAC)

- **Fig. 11: ETL utilizing retention suture for TAC.** The intra-abdominal edema and the abdominal wall necrosis underneath the retention suture plates are clearly visible. Severe abdominal wall necroses occur with this device. There is no reduction of intra-abdominal pressure. It should no longer be utilized.
- **Fig. 12: ETL utilizing a commercially available zipper for TAC.** The abdomen is open; the parietal peritoneum is inflamed. A plastic (polyethylene) drape is used to cover the bowel and omentum. There is no reduction of intra-abdominal pressure.
- **Fig. 13: ETL utilizing a glider (ETZIP®) for TAC.** The large sheaths allowing for abdominal expansion are clearly visible. The glider unfortunately can open spontaneously, leading to uncontrolled eventration.
- ETL utilizing the artificial burr for TAC. The abdomen

is closed. The hook sheet is on top of the sling sheet to which it adheres. Note the wide opening of the abdominal aperture (see p. 61).

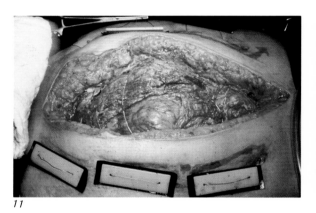

11

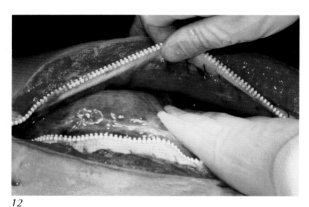

12

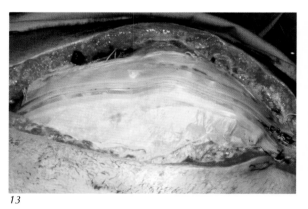

13

Of the four different methods for TAC, use of retention sutures (R-TAC) was associated with the majority of complications. It causes severe necroses of the abdominal wall. R-TAC and Z-TAC (simple zipper, Fig. 12) did not allow for decompression of the intra-abdominal pressure. The slide fastener or glider (G-TAC, Fig. 13) is large enough to permit intra-abdominal decompression, but may open when the patient moves in bed. This requires immediate re-operation. Another problem encountered with the zipper is its need to be replaced by one with a smaller seam once the inflammatory edema

subsides. These problems are avoided with the artificial burr. It enables gradual approximation of the fasciae along with the decrease of the inflammatory edema (Fig. 4), and removal and resuturing the device to the fascia is no more longer necessary.

Etappenlavage: Experience of Two Institutions

Beginning in 1980, Etappenlavage was performed at two institutions in 130 severely ill patients with diffuse peritonitis. During this period, these patients represented approximately

16% of all peritonitis cases. A total of 713 operations were necessary. The median duration from onset of signs of infection to initial ETL was 123 hours (63–300). Evidence of multiple-system organ failure was present in most patients. 57% of the infections were due to perforation of an intestinal viscus secondary to inflammation, obstruction, or other causes. 43% occurred postoperatively after abdominal surgery. 26% of these died. Mechanical ventilatory support was necessary for a median of 17 (3–90) days. 32 primary anastomoses were tolerated, with a mortality of 33%. During the lavage period, 61 additional complications placed by devices allowing for abdominal expansion without exerting increased intra-abdominal pressure. With these devices, forceful approximation of the abdominal fasciae was avoided, thus combining the concept of the open abdomen with that of the planned relaparotomies. Two authors, from Spain and Canada, published a paper that described a procedure in which the zipper closure was combined with Marlex® mesh, representing the fusion of these two concepts.

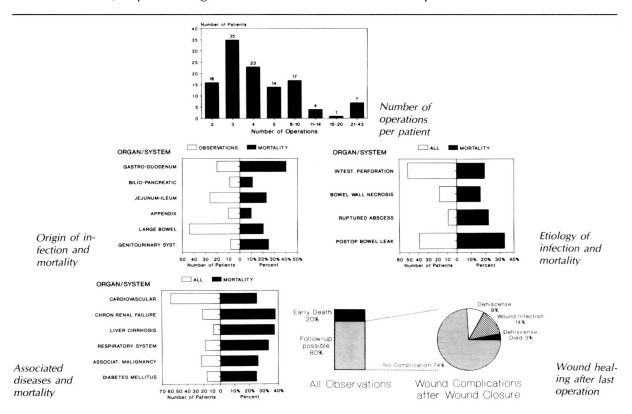

Number of operations per patient

Origin of infection and mortality

Etiology of infection and mortality

Associated diseases and mortality

Wound healing after last operation

were seen that required repair. Most patients had epidural anesthesia for a median of 9 (3–44) days, and the beginning of small bowel motility was observed during the lavage period in most cases.

The relatively low mortality (24%) in this high-risk group compares favorably with conventional surgical therapy and attests to its usefulness. The high-risk nature of the disease process in the ETL patients is not surprising given the additional risk factors of elderly patients, the relatively long duration of symptoms before treatment, and the high incidence of multiple-system organ failure in the patients of this series. Patients over the age of 70 had a mortality of 40%, indicating exhaustion of vital reserves in a special patient group. Postoperative peritonitis accounted for 42% of patients in this series. Postoperative peritonitis can carry a mortality ex-

ceeding 72%, and, given a mortality of 26% in ETL patients, there seems to be a particularly useful indication for ETL in postoperative peritonitis.

During the lavage period we discovered additional problems not seen at the first laparotomy; these might have been missed by closed operative techniques. Fistula formation as seen with the open-abdomen methods was not a problem in this series. ETL also allowed inspection of newly created anastomoses. The relatively low complication rate seen after definitive wound closure compares favorably to the open-abdomen technique. The majority of wound infections developed in patients who had fewer than five operations, indicating that local defense, as a function of time, may be more effective in older wounds. The ETL concept for diffuse peritonitis ensures improved elimination

of infectious source, better reduction of the bacterial inoculum in the peritoneal cavity, and better elimination of toxic necrotic material. With ETL, early diagnosis and therapy of postoperative complications are possible. ETL is a flexible therapeutic modality that avoids complications seen with intraperitoneal drains. The results reported here confirm the theoretical advantages discussed by Maddaus and Simmons: "Fluid, microbes and infection-potentiating agents are removed intermittently, persistent sepsis and intestinal leak or necrosis are detected early, fluid and protein losses are diminished, and it offers the possibility of evaluating the persistence or eradication of the infectious process." Final confirmation, however, might be obtained only from a controlled study. The most useful device for TAC has proved to be V-TAC the artificial burr.

Critical-Care Therapy

The objective of intensive- or critical-care therapy is threefold: 1) the regeneration of physiology, 2) the reduction of damage to all organ systems, and 3) the regulation of often excessive pathophysiological defense mechanisms.

Pulmonary Failure

Hypoxemia accompanying respiratory failure due to peritonitis is treated by artificial respiration with positive end-expiratory pressure (PEEP). This method improves oxygenation by increasing the functional residual capacity. It also reduces the intrapulmonary right-left shunt and improves compliance. To facilitate withdrawal from artificial respiration, intermittent mandatory ventilation (IMV), spontaneous respiration against increased end-expiratory pressure (CPAP), and other methods are adopted. Epidural analgesics also help to facilitate withdrawal.

Cardiovascular Failure

The stabilization of the circulatory system is just as important as the therapy of the pulmonary failure. Circulatory dysregulation occurring as a result of sepsis, fluid shifts, and artificial respiration requires continuous cardiocirculatory monitoring (arterial, venous, and pulmonary arterial capillary pressure measurement). Following placement of a Swan-Ganz thermodilution catheter, one can register an increased cardiac output often found during the early phase of sepsis. Not until the later stages of peritonitis does cardiac output decrease. At the first sign of a volume depletion (arterial hypotension, tachycardia with reduced filling pressure), crystalloid electrolyte solutions and especially such colloidal solutions as plasma, fresh blood, and human albumin are administered to replete intravascular volume. Dopamine and dobutamine provide pharmacological support of the circulatory system. In cases of pulmonary hypertension, nitroglycerin reduces the pre- and afterload.

Renal Failure

Renal failure accompanying peritonitis can be recognized as oliguria, an increase of urea and creatinine values, as well as by a shift in the urea-plasma osmolality quotient. The latter is a sure sign for the early stages of a shock kidney. According to studies by Lawrence and Weil, urine and plasma become isomolar as creatinine serum levels rise. Under these conditions the urea-plasma quotient equals 1. Under normal concentration conditions this quotient averages 1.6. Therapy is aimed primarily at the stabilization of the circulatory system, with volume repletion and the administration of dopamine to improve renal perfusion. In patients with acute renal impairment, early hemofiltration or hemodialysis is necessary to prevent complications such as hyperkalemia, hypervolemia, and reduction in pulmonary function, all of which compromise the healing chances of the patient.

Paralytic Ileus

Gastrointestinal atony with no peristalsis and significant loss of intestinal fluid are typical signs of paralytic ileus, often accompanying peritonitis. Via peridural anesthesia, cholinergics as well as sympatholytics can overcome the sympathetic-dependent blockage of intestinal motor responses.

Septic Shock

When local defense mechanisms are overpowered in the course of peritonitis, septic shock can result. Early diagnosis of this condition is important for rapid therapeutic treatment. Warning signals in laboratory diagnosis are thrombocytopenia, fibrinogen reduction, and lactic acidosis. In most cases, high doses of heparin can avoid intravascular coagulation. High doses of corticosteroids can favorably influence cell-membrane damage caused by endotoxins. Although septic shock has been shown to lower the IgG fraction, there is still no agreement on gammaglobulin therapy.

Diagnosis and Therapy of Peritonitis Complications	
Symptoms	Therapy
Pulmonary failure	
Hyperventilation Disturbed acid-base household Hypoxemia Functional residual capacity Compliance	Controlled artificial respiration with PEEP Weaning with IMV and CPAP Analgesia via epidural anaesthesia Reduction of intra-abdominal pressure using a broad device (e.g., artificial burr)
Hemodynamic failure	
Arterial hypotension Tachycardia Pulmonary hypertension Increased cardiac output (hyperdynamic state) and in the later phases decrease of cardiac (hypodynamic state) output	Volume substitution Dopamine Dobutamine Nitroglycerine (all measures monitor arterial and pulmonal-arterial pressure and control cardiac output)
Renal failure	
Oliguria: 30 ml/h Urea increase Creatinine increase $\dfrac{\text{Urine osmolality}}{\text{Plasma osmolality}} \leq 1.6$	Circulatory stabilization Dopamine Mannitol Early hemofiltration
Paralytic ileus	
Loss of liquids into the so-called "third space" Stomach-intestinal atonia (no peristalsis, loss of stomach fluids)	Sympathicolysis via epidural anaesthesia administered by a peridural catheter Cholinergics
Sepsis	
Hyperventilation Tachycardia, fever Hypotonia Thrombopenia Fibrinogen reduction Lactic acidemia	Heparin Cortisone? Switch to new antibiotics? Gammaglobulins? Physical measures Correction of acid-base disturbances

Antibiotic therapy of peritoneal inflammation begins under the conditions of a surgical emergency, i.e., prior to bacteriological results. Therefore, it must be directed against the various typical causative agents of peritonitis.

Most intra-abdominal infections require antibiotic therapy because surgical measures alone cannot eliminate the causative agents of infection. Antibiotic therapy should not begin until the diagnosis has been confirmed by laparotomy and infectious material has been removed for bacteriological analysis.

Chemotherapy initiated before the operation runs the risk of misdiagnosis. Moreover, the use of highly potent antibiotics may induce shock due to massive release of bacterial toxins from killed bacteria. In addition to the damage at hand, the operability of the patient would be further impaired. Furthermore, if antibiotic therapy is begun before the operation, it could prevent the comprehensive analysis of all pathogens responsible for the infection. In fact, the antibiotic drug could act on the infectious exudate during the transport in a test tube, for example, and thus destroy pathogens outside of the organism before they are grown on a culture. Gram-staining can only partially identify the pathogens responsible for abdominal inflammation.

In hospital situations where processing of the bacterial material cannot be performed within 10 minutes, many causative agents will die during transport procedures. Hence, it will not be possible to identify all pathogens. Under these circumstances, treatment proceeds without primary bacteriological evidence. As a rule, bacteriological investigation is to be pursued. At the same time, it is safe to say that most forms of peritonitis are caused by typical pathogen combinations. In individual cases, it is highly probable that such a bacterial spectrum causes the infection at hand; this allows for a calculated chemotherapy. Thus, the bacteria initially responsible for the infection are attacked.

However, should the symptoms of infection persist during the further course of the disease, maximum efforts must be made toward a qualitative bacteriological investigation. At hourly intervals three to six blood cultures must be placed in aerobic and anaerobic media capable of neutralizing antibiotics. Thus, pathogens are rapidly identified and, according to their sensitivity pattern, an antibiotic can be chosen to augment initial therapy.

Aminoglycosides are not suitable for the primary therapy of abdominal infections. As they are potentially nephrotoxic, the renal damage already initiated by the abdominal infection can be intensified and finally lead to renal failure, as has been shown in several controlled studies.

The initial antibiotic therapy need not be blind; rather, it should be calculated.

Is a directed antibiotic therapy possible?

NO !

Because an immediate identification of the causative agent by Gram-staining is not possible.	Because most of the bacteria die during sampling and transportation, making identification extremely difficult.
Because the antibiotic therapy must begin immediately after diagnosis.	Because it usually takes more than 2 days to obtain the results of sensitivity testing.

An antibiotic therapy directed against all pathogenetically significant agents is extremely difficult to realize under routine clinical conditions. The reasons for this are:
- Therapy must begin before the results of bacteriological investigations have been obtained.
- The isolation of pathogens creates technical difficulties, so many bacteria and their pathogenetic interactions remain undetected.
- The results of resistance tests are difficult to interpret and evaluate because the concentration levels of the antibiotics at the site of infection are not taken into account.

Insufficient data on the etiologically important pathogens and vague notions on their concentration-dependent activity at the site of infection characterize an antibiotic therapy that typically destroys only a few of the bacteria in the polymicrobial spectrum of peritonitis pathogens. But after the elimination of sensitive pathogens, primary resistant pathogens are then selected that lead to further damage in the peritonitis patient with weak defense.

An uncritical and too prolonged use of chemotherapeutics facilitates the formation of bacterial-resistance factors and their transfer from one bacterial species to another.

Calculated Antibiotic Therapy

The concept of a calculated antibiotic therapy was developed as a solution to the therapeutic dilemma of having to initiate chemotherapy of peritonitis in a state of "bacteriological blindness."

Calculated Antibiotic Therapy

- Is directed against a well-known typical spectrum of anaerobic and aerobic pathogens.
- Takes into consideration the various pathogenicity of causative agents and their synergistic and antagonistic interactions.
- Requires a sufficiently high concentration of antimicrobial medication at the site of infection.
- Has few side effects; in particular, it is not nephrotic.
- Does not infringe on the body's defenses beyond the traumatically conditioned degree.
- Is based on the results of clinically controlled studies.

Typical Pathogens

A calculated antibiotic therapy is a solution to the therapeutic difficulties stemming from the disguised results of routine pathogen isolation. The guiding hypothesis is that intra-abdominal infections are caused by a typical spectrum of pathogens since the causative agents are recruited from a single bacterial reservoir with relatively constant bacterial conditions. The basis for this hypothesis is the scientific examination of the bacterial patterns of a representative patient collective using optimal isolation techniques. These findings allow for generalizations as to the adequate therapeutic approach.

Indeed, as a comparison of a number of studies has shown, the pathogenic spectrum observed under such conditions in 900 cases of intra-abdominal infections shows a high congruence with respect to absolute and relative frequency of individual bacterial species. The analysis of the causative agents reveals an average of 2.9 pathogen species per infection. By definition, this is referred to as a mixed infection.

The complexity of mixed infections raises the question of therapy of the relevant target organism. The answer to this problem lies in a better understanding of the interactions between various pathogens and the interactions with adjuvants and with the body's own defense mechanisms.

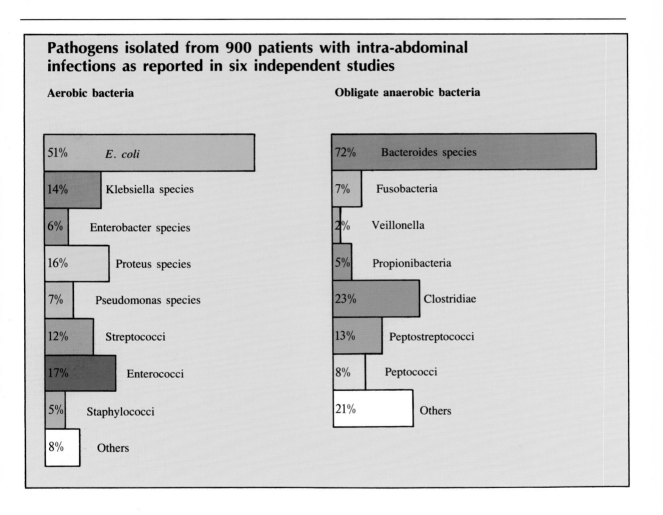

Pathogens isolated from 900 patients with intra-abdominal infections as reported in six independent studies

Aerobic bacteria

51% *E. coli*
14% Klebsiella species
6% Enterobacter species
16% Proteus species
7% Pseudomonas species
12% Streptococci
17% Enterococci
5% Staphylococci
8% Others

Obligate anaerobic bacteria

72% Bacteroides species
7% Fusobacteria
2% Veillonella
5% Propionibacteria
23% Clostridiae
13% Peptostreptococci
8% Peptococci
21% Others

Calculated Antibiotic Therapy

Bacterial pathogenicity factor =

$$Q = \frac{\text{Relative frequency in IAI}}{\text{Relative frequency in the intestines}}$$

The Pathogenicity of Causative Agents

The pathogenicity of individual infective agents can be expressed in terms of a comparison between the relative frequency of bacteria in the intestines and their relative distribution in intra-abdominal infections. Such a comparison reveals distinctive distribution patterns for various forms of peritonitis. Perforation, for example, represents the extreme case where the entire intestinal content reaches the free abdominal cavity.

The share of *E. coli* in the intestinal flora is less than 0.06%. However, this organism is found in 51% of the cases in intra-abdominal infections (pathogenicity factor Q = 850). This is an expression of the outstanding pathogenicity of *E. coli* in the infectious disease peritonitis.

Obligate anaerobic bacteria are typical for the intestinal flora and are virtually always found there (99%). In intra-abdominal infections they are isolated only immediately following perforation since they die rapidly outside the intestinal lumen. Thus, they can have no pathogenic effect on the organism.

The relative frequency of Bacteroides species in the intestines is 27%. The relative frequency of these organisms in intra-abdominal infections is only 1.3 times greater. Hence, they belong to the less pathogenic intestinal bacteria. But detailed analysis reveals that individual Bacteroides species differ considerably in their pathogenicity. In intra-abdominal infections, *Bacteroides melaninogenicus* is 100 times more frequent than in the intestines. Overall, however, its relative share of the intestinal flora is so small that it is relatively seldom seen in intra-abdominal infections. In the case of *Bacteroides fragilis,* the quotient of its relative frequency in intra-abdominal infections and in the intestines is 62. Although *B. fragilis* represents only 0.6% of the intestinal flora, it is the second most frequent pathogen causing intra-abdominal infections after *E. coli*. *B. fragilis* is thus an important target organism for therapy.

Other intestinal organisms qualifying as pathogens include Clostridiae (*C. perfringens* is the third most frequent pathogen), the enterobacteria belonging to the Klebsiella/Enterobacter group, and the Proteus species. The gram-positive chain cocci subsumed under the term *enterococci* are found 130 times more frequently in intra-abdominal infections than in the intestines. The other aerobic streptococci are found 600 times more frequently in intra-abdominal infections (see t. on page 69). *Pseudomonas aeruginosa* and staphylococci play a subordinate role in intra-abdominal infections.

In effect, *E. coli, Bacteroides fragilis,* and Clostridiae represent the most important target organisms for therapy in intra-abdominal infections. Since intra-abdominal infections are mixed infections, an understanding of synergistic effects between various pathogens is important for interpreting the progress of the infection and choosing a therapeutic strategy.

70

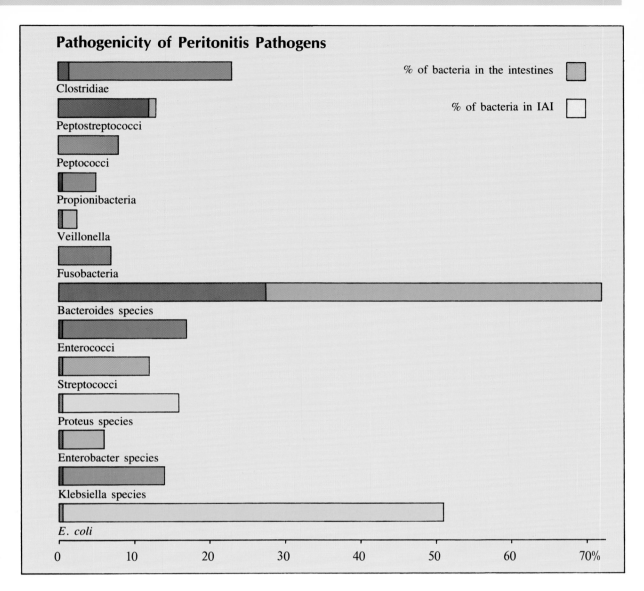

Pathogenicity of Peritonitis Pathogens

% of bacteria in the intestines

% of bacteria in IAI

Clostridiae

Peptostreptococci

Peptococci

Propionibacteria

Veillonella

Fusobacteria

Bacteroides species

Enterococci

Streptococci

Proteus species

Enterobacter species

Klebsiella species

E. coli

0 10 20 30 40 50 60 70%

Bacterial Synergism

The synergistic effects of various bacterial species can be studied in animal models. In general, the results of animal experiments are limited in their value in explaining the total picture of intraabdominal infections in humans, where a multitude of factors related to both the patient and the therapy influence the course of the disease. Still, experiments with the implantation of feces in the animal abdomen correlate with the clinical progress of the disease in humans (see pp. 30–31).

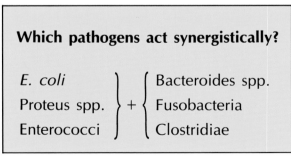

Which pathogens act synergistically?

E. coli
Proteus spp. } + { Bacteroides spp.
Enterococci   Fusobacteria
                 Clostridiae

Adjuvants

An understanding of the toxic and infection-promoting effects of adjuvants such as bile, mucus, hemoglobin, certain components of feces, and barium sulfate are especially important for operative therapy (p. 33).

Calculated Antibiotic Therapy

The primary aim of antibiotic therapy is to combat the infection at the site of infection and not solely in the circulation.

Antibiotic Concentration at the Site of Infection

To successfully combat infection at its site, the primary aim of antibiotic therapy, the results of studies on the concentration dynamics of antimicrobial substances at the site of infection must be taken into account. These studies have shown that peritoneal exudate is a bodily fluid that represents the site of infection in intra-abdominal infections. Moreover, this fluid allows for reproducible measurements of antibiotic concentrations following intravenous administration. Peritoneal exudate is formed by inflamed tissue. Via peritoneal stomata of the diaphragm and thoratic lymph channels, 80% of this liquid enters the venous bloodstream. The chemical composition of the peritoneal exudate is similar to that of the thoracic lymph.

The antibiotic concentration that is active at the site of infection is expressed as the evaluative concentration ϵ (= C_{eff}). As a function of concentration level and the duration of the concentration level, ϵ is time-dependent As with precisely calculated minimum inhibitory concentrations in the laboratory, this assures irreversible destruction of the pathogens at the site of infection.

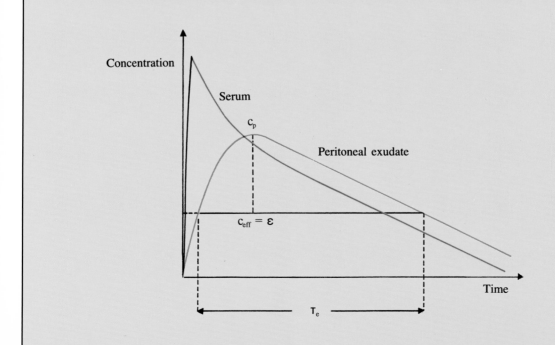

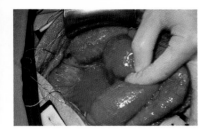

Antimicrobial concentration measured in peritoneal fluid is representative for the site of infection in peritonitis

Interactions between Antibiotics and Host Defense System

Many antibiotics have been shown to interact with the organism either as an immunostimulant or, in part, as a depressant of the cellular and humoral immune response. Studies of both have led to conflicting observations. At present, it is difficult to derive any recommendation for therapy.

Side Effects of Antibiotics

Today's antibiotics are characterized by extremely low toxicity and side-effect rates in relation to their therapeutic activity. In the management of peritonitis, the potential nephrotoxicity of antibiotics plays an important role. This has been shown by several controlled studies of peritonitis patients in whom the renal system is often already compromised.

Results of Controlled Clinical Studies: Bias or Truth?

The superiority of a given therapy can ultimately be demonstrated only by controlled studies comparing homogeneous patient populations. In particular, new antibiotics should not be employed in routine practice until they have been tested in neat randomized, controlled studies with well-defined patient groups and so demonstrated their therapeutic superiority. Controlled studies comparing different antibiotic regimen for peritonitis, however, are strongly prebiased; i.e., the study design precludes valuable clinical information. Joe Solomkin, in a very thorough overview, was able to show this phenomenon for intra-abdominal infections. In controlled studies sponsored by pharmaceutical companies, patients of clinical concern were excluded from the studies, resulting in a overall mortality of 3.5%. This is in strong contrast to a 10-fold higher mortality in real life. Consequently, prospective controlled studies looking at antibiotic efficacy in peritonitis are not of any help in clinical decision making, and must be interpreted with great caution. Bacteriological and pharmacological data, on this background, regain relative importance.

As a rule of thumb and keeping the severity of infection in mind, the following measures against side effects of antibiotics should be considered:

Side effect	Measure
Nephrotoxicity	No aminoglycosides
Bleeding	Vitamin K replacement
Disturbed hematopoiesis	Change of drugs
Allergy	Anamnestic evaluation

The data compiled in this book reflect the complex picture of intra-abdominal infections with their many pathogenetic factors and therapeutic possibilities. In light of the many factors involved, it seems virtually impossible to state a general, scientifically based recommendation for therapy. Yet clinical practice demands quick decisions and ac-

Objective?

As discussed in the previous chapters, the chemotherapy of peritonitis begins without knowledge of the pathogens responsible for individual cases. Hence, the treatment must be directed against a bacterial spectrum that has been isolated from many patients with the respective primary disease and that can thus be considered typical of the disease.

The essential target organisms are those forming endotoxins, in particular, *E. coli.* A second group of target organisms, namely anaerobic bacteria, must also be taken into account during the initial therapy. Enterococci must be considered if obligate anaerobic organisms are not covered by the antimicrobial spectrum. *Pseudomonas aeruginosa* and *Staphylococcus aureus* play a subordinate role.

Adjuvants (see p. 33) must be surgically removed as far as possible. In the course of surgery, the bacterial count must be reduced to an inoculum susceptible to antibiotic treatment. In other words, the source of infection must be removed and new sources of infection or an insufficiency of the suture for the primary source of infection must be avoided. This can be achieved by means of etappen-lavage.

Intensive care sets the stage for operative procedures and repairs damage already present. In the future, we need a better understanding of the effects of various toxins produced by bacterial species.

tions, however variable the basic parameters may be. Therapy recommendations must be viewed relative to these reservations.

Timing?

Antibiotic therapy deals with only a few toxic substances in conjunction with the operation. Based on a fixed diagnosis immediately after opening the abdominal cavity, large masses of bacteria are surgically removed from the abdomen.

If the symptoms of infection do not recede within 3 days, a qualitatively sensitive bacteriological analysis is necessary to isolate from the blood those pathogens responsible for the persistence of infection symptoms. At this point, three to six blood cultures must be sampled at hourly intervals and bacteriologically processed as fast as possible. The samples must be taken under aerobic and anaerobic conditions—if necessary, using an antibiotic-removing device (ARD).

In individual cases, it is advisable to discontinue administration of the antibiotics that are therapeutically not fully effective. This assures that the aspirated blood in the culture flasks does not contain antibiotics that are possibly more active against bacteria in vitro than in vivo. In any case, samples of such blood cultures must be taken at the end of a dose interval, immediately before administration of the next dose, so that the blood culture contains a minimal concentration of antibiotics.

Medication?

The calculated antibiotic therapy is directed against target organisms. The most important target organisms are *E. coli* and *Bacteroides fragilis,* as well as Clostridiae. Third-generation cephalosporins such as cefotaxime in combination with an imidazole preparation such as metronidazole are especially effective against these etiologically important pathogens.

Procedure?

Antibiotic therapy should be systemic and not local. Following systemic administration, preferably a bolus injection, reproducible antibiotic concentrations are achieved at the site of infection. Local therapy presents the risk of nonuniform antibiotic concentrations at the site of injection. This promotes the selection of resistant bacteria and can lead to unreliable treatment results. The effectiveness of local therapeutic treatment has not been sufficiently documented by controlled clinical studies.

Bibliography

Allen L. The peritoneal stomata. The Anatomical Report 67:89–103, 1936.

Allen L, Wetherford T. Role of penetrated basement in lymphatic absorbation from peritoneal cavity. Am J Physiol 197:551–554, 1959.

Altemeier WA. Perspectives in Surgical Infections. Surg Clin North Am 60:5–13, 1980.

Altemeier WA. The bacterial flora of acute perforated appendicitis with peritonitis. Ann Surg 107:517–528, 1938.

Altemeier WA. The cause of the putrid odor of perforated appendicitis with peritonitis. Ann Surg 107:634–636, 1938.

Altemeier WA. The pathogenicity of the bacteria of appendicitis peritonitis. Surgery 11:374–384, 1942.

Altemeier WA. Surgical infection of the peritoneum. Surg Clin North Am 22:437–454, 1942.

Altemeier WA, Culbertson WR, Fullen WD, Shook CD. Intra-abdominal abscesses. Am J Surg 125:70–79, 1973.

Altunbay S, Bleiler HJ, Heil H. Die postoperative Peritonitis. Fortschr Med 100:560–565, 1982.

Anders A. Die sekundäre Peritonitis. In: P Kempf (ed): Behandlung der Peritonitis. Zuckschwerdt, Munich, 1980, pp 167–175.

Anderson E, Mandelbaum DM, Ellison EC. Open packing of the peritoneal cavity in generalized bacterial peritonitis. Am J Surg 145:131–135, 1983.

Andrus C, Doering M, Herrmann VM, Kaminski DL. Planned reoperation of generalized intra-abdominal infection. Am J Surg 152:682–686, 1986.

Arbeitsgemeinschaft Peritonitis: Bakteriologische Befunde bei verschiedenen Peritonitisformen. In: DH Wittmann (ed): Intraabdominelle Infektionen. Fortschr Antimikrob Antineoplast Chemother (FAC) Bd. 2–3. Futuramed, Munich, 1983, pp 423–429.

Aune S. Transperitoneal exchange. Scand J Gastroenterol 5:85–99, 1970.

Autio V. The spread of intraperitoneal infection. Studies with roentgen contrast medium. Acta chir 131(Suppl):1–31, 1964.

Bartels H, Lehr L, Gubernales G, Hlscher N. Die programmierte Relaparotomie als Therapiekonzept bei der diffusen 4-Quadranten-SE Peritonitis.

Langenbecks Arch 366:631–632, 1985.

Bartlett JG. Anaerobes in human inection. In: SM Finegold (ed): Metronidazole. Proceedings of the International Metronidazole Conference Montreal. Excerpta Medica, Amsterdam, 1976, pp 261–270.

Bartlett JG. Interdependence and synergism in anaerobic infection. In: I Phillips, J Collier (eds): Metronidazole. The Royal Society of Medicine, Academic Press, London, 1979, pp 7–12.

Bartlett JG. Lesson on intra-abdominale sepsis from an animal model. Proc Symp: The Use of Beta-Lactam Antibiotics in Gynecological and Surgical Infections. Indiana University School of Medicine, Chicago, 1983.

Bartlett JG, Miao PVW, Gorbach SL: Empiric treatment with clindamycin and gentamicin of suspected sepsis due to anaerobic and aerobic bacteria. J Infect Dis 135(Suppl):80, 1977.

Bauernfeind A, Wittmann DH. Erregerspezifische Pathogenitätsfaktoren der Mikroflora bei Peritonitiden. In: DH Wittmann (ed): Intraabdominelle Infektionen. Fortschr Antimikrob Antineoplast Chemother (FAC) Bd 2–3. Futuramed, Munich, 1983, pp 431–436.

Becker HD, Boerger HW, Schafmeyer A. Operationstaktik und -technik bei Peritonitis nach Oberbaucheingriffen. Langenbecks Arch Chir 352:311–316, 1980.

Beger HG, Kraas E, Bittner R. Endotoxinschock: Erkennung und Behandlung. Langenbecks Arch Chir 352:307–310, 1980.

Beger HG, Gogler H, Kraas E, Bittner R. Endotoxin bei bakterieller Peritonitis. Chirurg 52:81–88, 1981.

Bergey's Manual of Determinative Bacteriology. 8th Ed, Baltimore, 1974. Vol I: International Code of Nomenclature of Bacteria. Washington, DC, 1975.

Braun L, Santger R, Michalke HJ. Die fortgeschrittene Peritonitis. Beitr Klin Chir 221:120–128, 1974.

Broome A, Hansson L, Lundgren F. Open treatment of abdominal septic catastrophies. World J Surg 7:792–796, 1983.

Bruchard KW, Ciombor DM, McLeod MK, Slothman GJ, Gann DS. Positive end expiratory pressure with increased intra-abdominal pressure. Surg

Gyn Obstet 161:313–318, 1985.

Brütt H. Die Bedeutung der anaeroben Streptokokken für die destruktive Appendizitis. Beitr Klin Chir 129:175–185, 1923.

Burke J. The physiology of wound infection. In: TK Hunt (ed): Wound Healing and Wound Infection. Appleton-Century-Crofts, New York, 1980, pp 242–249.

Cain JL, Labat JA, Cohn Jr J. Bile peritonitis in germ-free dogs. Gastroenterol 53:600–608, 1967.

Caselitz F-H, Freitag V. Halbflüssiges Kombinationsnährmedium (TVLS-Medium) zur Züchtung anaerober Bakterien. Arztl Lab 15:426–430, 1969.

Champault G, Magnier U, Psalmon F et al. L'éviscération "contrôlée" dans le traitement des péritonites graves. Chirurgie 106:866–869, 1979.

Chellappa M. Peritonitis in southeast Asia region. In: DH Wittmann, JS Solomkin (eds): International Congress on Intraabdominal Infections, Hamburg, 1987.

Christou NV. Systemic and peritoneal host defense in peritonitis. World J Surg 14:184–190, 1990.

Clarke JS, Bartlett JG, Finegold SM, Gorbach SL, Wilson SE. Bacteriology of the gut and its clinical implications. West J Med 212:390–403, 1974.

Collee JG. Mechanisms of pathogenicity of anaerobic bacteria of clinical interest. Infection 8(Suppl):113–117, 1980.

Collee JL. Factors contributing to loss of anaerobic bacteria in transit from the patient to laboratory. Infection 8(Suppl):145–147, 1980.

Condon RE. Management of the acute complications of diverticular disease. Dis Colon Rectum 19:296–300, 1976.

Condon RE: Peritonitis and intraabdominal abscess. In: SI Schwartz, GT Shires, FC Spender, EH Storer (eds): Principles of Surgery. 1979, pp 1398–1423.

Conn H, Fessel M: Spontaneous bacterial peritonitis in cirrhosis: variations on a theme. Medicine 50:161, 1971.

Courtice FC. Lymph and plasma proteins: barriers to their movement throughout the extracellular fluid. Lymphology 4:9–17, 1971.

Courtice FC, Simmonds WJ. Physiological significance of lymph drainage of the serous cavities and lung. Physiol Rev 34:419–448, 1954.

Courtice FC, Steinbeck AW. Absorption of protein from the peritoneal cavity. J Physiol 114:336–355, 1951.

Cullen DJ, Coyle JP, Teplick R, Long MC. Cardiovascular, pulmonary, and renal effects of massively increased intra-abdominal pressure in critically ill patients. Crit Care Med 17:118–121, 1989.

Daschner F. Probleme der antibakteriellen Lokaltherapie. In: C Burri, A Rüter (eds): Lokalbehandlung chirurgischer Infektionen. Huber, Bern, 1979, pp 18–21.

Dellinger EP, Wertz MJ, Meakins JL: Surgical infection stratification system for intra-abdominal infection. Arch Surg 120:21, 1985.

Desa LA, Metha SJ, Nadkarni KM, Bhalero RA. Peritonitis: A study of factors contributing to mortality. Indian J Surg 45:593–603

Deutsches Institut für Normung e.V. Methoden zur Empfindlichkeitsprüfung von bakteriellen Krankheitserregern außer Mycobakterien gegenüber Chemotherapeutika. DIN 58940. Beuth, Berlin, 1982.

Dinstl K. Die Spübehandlung der Peritonitis. In: R Häring (ed): Peritonitis. TM-Verlag, Bad Oeynhausen, 1979, pp 123–126.

Dittrich H. Wundheilungsstörungen. Chirurg 42:289–295, 1971.

Doutre LP, Perissat J, Sarire, et al. La Laparostomie: methode d'exception dans le traitement des peritonites gravissimes. A propos de 29 observations. Bordeaux Med 15:195, 1982.

Duff JH, Moffat J. Abdominal sepsis managed by leaving abdomen open. Surgery 90:774–778, 1981.

Duff JH, Groves AC, McLean AP, LaPointe ER, McLean LD. Defective oxygen consumption in septic shock. Surg Gynec Obstet 128:1051–1060, 1969.

Dumont AE. The flow capacity of the thoracic duct venous junction. Am J Med Sci 269:292–301, 1975.

Eckert P, Eichfuss, HP. Peritonitis. Thieme, Stuttgart, 1978.

Edmiston CE, Goheen MP, Kornhall S, et al. Fecal peritonitis: Microbial adherence to serosal mesothelium and resistance to peritoneal lavage. World J Surg 14:176–183, 1990.

Eggert A, Freitag V, Schimmel G, Wittmann DH. Zur Technik der intraoperativen Diagnostik von Gallenweginfektionen. Arztl Lab 25:79–82, 1979.

Enander L-K, Nilson F, Ryden A-C, Schawan A. The aerobic and anaerobic microflora of the gastric remnant more than 15 years after Billroth II. Scand J Gastroenterol 17:715–720, 1982.

Enke A, Boetcher W. Das Vorgehen bei Perforationsperitonitis, Vorbereitung und Zeitpunkt der Operation. Langenbecks Arch Chir 349:495–498, 1979.

Esser G, Rappen HH. Über die Effektivität der Spüldrainagen bei diffuser bakterieller Peritonitis. Chirurg 51:774–776, 1980.

Fagniez PL. La prévention des lésions intestinales lors de éviscerations. Nouv Presse Méd 7:1117, 1978.

Fagniez PL, Hay JM, Regnier B, et al. Les peritonites "depasses." Attitudes therapeutique et resultats. Nouv Presse Méd 8:1348–1349, 1979.

Famos M. Peritonitis-Index. Vortrag bei der III. Tagung der Arbeitsgemeinschaft Peritonitis. Frankfurt, May 17, 1985.

Farthmann EH, Schöffel U. Principles and limitations of operative management of intra-abdominal infections. World J Surg 14:210–217, 1990.

Farthmann EH, Lehberger FJ, Knauf M, Pulvermüller A. Die postoperative Peritonitis. In: R Häring (ed): Peritonitis, TM-Verlag, Bad Oeynhausen, 1979, pp 181–186.

Finegold SM. Anaerobic bacteria in human disease. Academic Press, New York, 1977.

Finegold SM. Microflora of the gastrointestinal tract. In: SE Wilson, SM Finegold, RA Williams (eds): Intra-abdominal Infection, McGraw-Hill, New York, 1982, pp 1–22.

Fleming A. On the antibacterial action of cultures of a penicillium, with special reference to their use in the isolation of b. influenzae. Br J Exp Pathol 10:226–236, 1929.

Friedrich PL. Zur bacteriellen Aetiologie und zur Behandlung der diffusen Peritonitis. Arch Klin Chir 68:524–527, 1902.

Fromkes JJ, Thomas-Mekhjian HS, Evans M. Antimicrobial activity of human ascitic fluid.

Gastroenterology 73:668–672, 1977.

Fry DE, Pearlstein L, Fulton RL, Polk HC Jr. Multiple system organ failure: the role of uncontrolled infection. Arch Surg 115:136–140, 1981.

Gall F. Frühzeitige Relaparotomie bei Peritonitis, intraabdominellen Abszessen und Dünndarmfisteln. Langenbecks Arch Klin Chir 313:175–189, 1965.

Garcia-Sabrido JL, Quintans A, Polo JR. Lavado peritoneal postoperatorio continuo (LPPC) en peritonitis de alto riesgo (PAR). Cir Esp 39:73–76, 1985.

Garcia-Sabrido JM, Tallado JM, Christou NV. Treatment of severe intra-abdominal sepsis and/or necrotic foci by an "open-abdomen" approach. Zipper and zipper-mesh techniques. Arch Surg 123:152–156, 1988.

Gjessing J, Tomlin P. Continuous peritoneal lavage. Acta Chir Scand 140:124–129, 1974.

Goertz G. Die Wirkung einer intraoperativen Bauchhöhlenwaschung mit verschiedenen Antiseptica bei experimenteller Peritonitis. Langenbecks Arch Chir (Suppl):177–183, 1982.

Goertz G, Häring R. Die Peritonitis als Infektionsmodell. In: DH Wittmann (ed): Intraabdominelle Infektionen. Fortschr Antimikrob Antineoplast Chemother (FAC) Bd 2–3. Futuramed, Munich, 1983, pp 447–458.

Gonzenbach HR, Sonnabend W. Moxalactam—ein neues β-Lactam Antibiotikum in Monotherapie bei schweren Infektionskrankheiten in der Chirurgie. Schweiz Med Wschr 31/32:1, 1981.

Gorbach SL. Normal bowel flora and intra-abdominal sepsis in bacteriology of the gut and its clinical implication. West J Med 121:390, 1974.

Gorbach SL, Bartlett JG. Anaerobic infections. N Engl J Med 290:1177–1184, 1237–1245, 1280–1291, 1974.

Gorbach SL, Nahas L, Lerner P, Weinstein L. Studies of intestinal microflora: I. Effects of age, diet, and periodic sampling on numbers of fecal microorganisms in man. Gastroenterology 53:845–855, 1967.

Gorbach SL, Plaut AC, Nahas L, Weinstein L. Studies of intestinal microflora: II. Microorganisms of the small intestine and their relations to oral and

Bibliography

fecal flora. Gastroenterology 53:856–873, 1967.

Goris RJA. Ogilvie's method applied to infected wound disruption. Arch Surg 115:1103–1107, 1980.

Goris RJA, Boekhorst TPA, Nuytinck JKS, et al. Multiple organ failure: Generalized autodestructive inflammation? Arch Surg 120:1109–1115, 1985.

Greenlee HB, Gelbart SM, DeOrio AJ, Francescatti DS, Paez J, Reinhardt GF. The influence of gastric surgery on the intestinal flora. Am J Clin Nutrit 30:1826–1833, 1977.

Guivarc'h M, Roullet-Audy JC, Chapman A. La non fermeture pariétale dans la chirurgie itérative des péritonites. Chirurgie 105:287–290, 1979.

Haaga JR. Imaging intra-abdominal abscesses and nonoperative drainage procedures. World J Surg 14:204–209, 1990.

Hagen JC, Wood WS, Hashimoto T. In vitro stimulation of *Bacteroides fragilis* growth by *Escherichia coli*. Eur J Clin Microbiol 1:338–343, 1982.

Halbfass HJ, Keller H, Boesken WH. Ergebnisse der kontinuierlichen Dauerspülung bei diffuseitriger Peritonitis. Chirurg 53:628–632, 1982.

Haljamae H. Anatomy of the interstitial tissue. Lymphology 11:128–132, 1978.

Häring R. Peritonitis. In: R Häring (ed): Dringliche Bauchchirurgie. Thieme, Stuttgart, 1982, pp 56–112.

Hau T. Bacteria, toxins and the peritoneum. World J Surg 14:167–175, 1990.

Hau T, Ahrenholz DH, Simmons RL. Secondary bacterial peritonitis: The biologic basis of treatment. In: Current problems in Surgery. Vol 14(I). Year Book Medical Publishers, Chicago, 1979, pp 5–65.

Hay JM, Duchatelle P, Elman A, Flamant Y, Maillard JN. Les ventres laissés ouverts. Chirurgie 105:508–510, 1979.

Heddrich GS, Wexler MJ, McLean APH, Meakins JL. The septic abdomen: open management with Marlex mesh with a zipper. Surgery 99:399–408, 1986.

Heinrich S, Pulverer G. Über den Nachweis des Bacteroides melaninogenicus in Krankheitsprozessen bei Mensch und Tier. Zeitschr Hyg 146:331–340, 1960.

Herfarth Ch, Heil Th. Therapeutische Richtlinien bei postoperativer Peritonitis und Reintervention (Antibiotika, Drainage, Spülung). Langenbecks Arch Chir 352:301–306, 1980.

Heyde M. Bakteriologische und experimentelle Untersuchungen zur Atiologie der Wurmfortsatzentzündung mit besonderer Berücksichtigung anaerober Bakterien. Beitr Klin Chir 76:1–12, 1911.

Hite KE, Locke M, Hesseltine HC. Synergism in experimental infections with nonsporulating anaerobic bacteria. J Infect Dis 84:1–9, 1949.

Hollender LF, Bur F, Schwenk D, Pigache P. Das "offengelassene Abdomen." Technik, Indikation, Resultate. Chirurg 54:316–319, 1983.

Hugh TB, Nankivell C, Meagher AP, Li B. Is closure of the peritoneal layer necessary in the repair of midline surgical abdominal wounds? World J Surg 14:231–234, 1990.

Hunt JL. Generalized peritonitis. To irrigate or not to irrigate the abdominal cavity. Arch Surg 117:209–212, 1982.

Jansen HH. Peritonitis aus pathologisch-anatomischer Sicht. Leber-Magen-Darm 11:167–173, 1981.

Jeckstadt P, Wittmann DH. Index zur Beurteilung der Prognose intraabdomineller Infektionen. In: DH Wittmann (ed): Intraabdominelle Infektionen. Fortschr Antimikrob Antineoplast Chemother (FAC) Bd 2–3. Futuramed, Munich, 1983, pp 517–524.

Kaene FW, Everett ED, Fine RN, et al. CAPD related peritonitis management and antibiotic therapy recommendations. Peritoneal Dial Bull 7:55, 1987.

Kern E, Klaue P, Arbogast R. Programmierte Peritoneal-Lavage bei diffuser Peritonitis. Chirurg 54:306–310, 1983.

Kerremanns R, Pennickx F, et al. Mortality of diffuse peritonitis patients reduced by planned relaparotomies. Inensivmed Notfallmed Anaesthesiol 37:104–107, 1982.

Kiene S, Troeger H. Intraperitoneale Antibiotica-Spüldrainage bei diffuser Peritonitis. Zbl Chir 99:833–840, 1974.

King CD, Toskes PP. Small intestinal bacterial overgrowth. Gastroenterology 76:1035–1055, 1979.

Kirschner M. Die Behandlung der akuten eitrigen freien Bauchfellentzündung. Langenbecks Arch Klin Chir 142:53–267, 1926.

Knaus WA, Draper EA, Wagner DP, Zimmerman JE. APACHE II: A severity of disease classification system. Crit Care Med 13:818–829, 1985.

Körte W. Erkrankungen und Verletzungen des Peritoneums. In: E von Bergmann, P von Bruns (eds): Handbuch der praktischen Chirurgie. Bd III: Chirurgie des Bauches. Thieme, Stuttgart, 1907.

Körte W. (quoted in Schmidt, 1941).

Kunz H. Die Peritonitis als Ursache postoperativer Todesfälle. Langenbecks Arch Klin Chir 313:170–173, 1965.

Kunz H. Drainage der Bauchhöhle. In: G Brant, H Kunz, R Nissen (eds): Intra- und postoperative Zwischenfälle. Bd II: Abdomen. Thieme, Stuttgart, 1965.

Lawrence WJ, Weil MH. Water, creatinine and sodium excretion following circulatory shock with renal failure. Am J Med 51:314, 1971.

Lazarou SA, Barbul A, Wasserkrug HL, Efron G. The wound is a possible source of post-traumatic immune suppression. Program, 9th Annual Meeting of the Surgical Infection Society, Denver, 1989.

Leguit P. Zip-closure of the abdomen. Neth J Surg 34:40–41, 1982.

Levy E. Principles of surgery for diffuse peritonitis. Management of the abdominal wall. (In French.) Ann Chir 39:547–553, 1985.

Lierse W. Das Peritoneum. Anatomische Grundlagen. Der Chirurg 56:357–361, 1985.

Linder MM, Ott W, Wesch G, Wicki O, Marti MC, Moser G. Die Behandlung der eitrigen Bauchfellentzündung. Untersuchungen des Krankengutes und Erfahrung mit dem neuen Chemotherapeutikum und Antiendotoxin Taurolin. Langenbecks Arch Chir 353:241–250, 1981.

Linder MM, Wacha H. Der Peritonitis-Index—Grundlage zur Bewertung der Peritonitis-Erkrankung? In: DH Wittmann (ed): Intraabdominelle Infektionen. Fortschr Antimikrob Antineoplast Chemother (FAC) Bd 2–3. Futuramed, Munich, 1983, pp 511–516.

Linzenmeier G. Experimentelle Infektionen durch anaerobe Sporenbildner (Clostridien) der

Gasbrandgruppe. In: O Eichler, A Farah, H Herken, AD Welch (eds): Handbuch der experimentellen Pharmakologie. Bd XVI (10). Springer, Berlin, 1966, pp 243–291.

Loehr W. Erfahrungen mit der Serumbehandlung der Peritonitis. Arch Klin Chir 197:283–318, 1939.

Loehr W, Raβfeld L. Die Bakteriologie der Wurmfortsatzentzündung und der appendiculären Peritonitis. Thieme, Leipzig, 1931.

Lorber B, Swenson RM. The bacteriology of intraabdominal infections. Surg Clin North Am 55:1349–1354, 1975.

Lorenz W. Rundtischgespräch: Die prospektive Studie. Methode zur Ermittlung des Therpieerfolges. Langenbecks Arch Chir 347:487–490, 1978.

Lorenz W, Rohde H. Prospective kontrollierte Studien in der Chirurgie. Klin Wschr 57:310, 1979.

Louie TJ, Onderdonk AB, Gorbach SL, Bartlett JG. Therapy for experimental intraabdominal sepsis of four cephalosporins with clindamycin plus gentamycin. J Infect Dis 135:S18–22, 1977.

Maddaus MA, Simmons RL. Leave the abdomen open for peritonitis: yes, no, maybe? Adv Surg 21:1–18, 1987.

Maetani S, Tobe T. Open peritoneal drainage as effective treatment of advanced peritonitis. Surgery 90:804–809, 1981.

Mastboom WJB, Kuypers HHC, Schoots FJ, Wobbes T. Small-bowel perforation complicating the open treatment of generalized peritonitis. Arch Surg 124:689–692, 1989.

McKenna JP, Currie DJ, MacDonald JA, et al. The use of continuous postoperative peritoneal lavage in the management of diffuse peritonitis. Surg Gynecol Obstet 130:254–280, 1970.

Meleney FL, Harvey HD, Jern HZ. Peritonitis. I. The correlation of the bacteriology of the peritoneal exudate and the clinical course of disease in 106 cases of peritonitis. Arch Surg 22:1–26, 1931.

Meleney FL, Ollp J, Harvey HD, Zaytseff-Jern H. Peritonitis: II. Synergism of bacteria commonly found in peritoneal exudates. Arch Surg 25:709–721, 1932.

Michaelis J. Kontrollierte Therapiestudien. Dtsch Med Wschr 107:1947–1950, 1982.

Mikulicz J. Über die Anwendung der Antisepsis bei Laparotomien mit besonderer Rücksicht auf die Drainage der Bauchhöhle. Arch Klin Chir 26:111–117, 1881.

Miles AA. Nonspecific defense reactions in bacterial infections. Ann NY Acad Sci 66:356–369, 1966.

Moore WEC. Anerobes as normal flora: gastrointestinal tract. In: SM Finegold (ed): Metronidazole. Proceedings of the International Metronidazole Conference Montreal. Excerpta Medica, Amsterdam, 1976, pp 222–228.

Moore WEC, Cato EP, Holdemann LV. Anaerobic bacteria of the gastrointestinal flora and their occurrence in clinical infections. J Infect Dis 119:641–649, 1969.

Mughal M, Bancewicz J, Irving MH. 'Laparoscopy." A technique for the management of intractable intra-abdominal sepsis. Br J Surg 73:253–259, 1986.

Muhrer KH, Grimm B, Wagner KH, Borner U. Serum-EndotoxinSpiegel wahrend des Verlaufs der offenen peritonitis behandlung. Chirurg 56:789–797, 1985.

Nichols RL, Smith JW. Intragastric microbial colonization in common disease states of the stomach and duodenum. Ann Surg 182:557–561, 1975.

Nichols RL, Smith JW, Balthazar ER. Peritonitis and intraabdominal abscess: an experimental model for the evaluation of human disease. J Surg Res 25:129–134, 1978.

Nichols WW, Crow MR, Nichols K. Diagnostic of anaerobic infection by gas chromatographic estimation of volatile fatty acids. Europ J Clin Microbiol 1:344–350, 1982.

Nyström PO, Bax R, Dellinger EP, et al: Proposed definitions for diagnosis, severity scoring, stratification and outcome for trials on intra-abdominal infection. World J Surg 14:148–156, 1990.

Ochsner A, DeBakey M. Subphrenic abscess: Collective review and analysis of 3608 collected and personal cases. Int Abst Surg 66:726–759, 1938.

Offenbartl K, Bengmark S. Intra-abdominal infections and gut origin sepsis. World J Surg 14:191–195, 1990.

Onderdonk A, Weinstein W, Sullivan NM, Bartlett JG, Gorbach SL. Experimental intraabdominal abscesses in rats: quantitative bacteriology of infected animals. Infect Immunol 10:1256–1259, 1974.

Onderdonk AB, Barlett JG, Louie T, Sullivan-Siegler N, Gorbach SL. Microbial synergy in experimental intraabdominal abscess. Infect Immunol 13:22–26, 1976.

Onderdonk AB, Kasper DL, Cisneros BL, Barlett JG. The capsular polysaccharide of Bacteroides fragilis as a virulence factor: comparison of the pathogenic potential of encapsulated and unencapsulated strains. J Infect Dis 136:82–89, 1977.

Onderdonk AB, Kaspar DL, Mansheim BJ, Louie TJ, Gorbach SL, Bartlett JG. Experimental animal models for anaerobic infections. Rev Infect Dis 1:291–301, 1979.

Penninckx FM, Kerremans RP, Lauwers PM. Planned relaparotomies in the surgical treatment of severe generalized peritonitis from intestinal origin. World J Surg 7:762–766, 1983.

Petermann J. Zur Behandlung der akuten diffusen Bauchfellentzündung. Med Welt 1:915–916, 1939.

Peters H, Zilkens KW. The importance of anaerobic infections in abdominal surgery. Infection 8:S192–193, 1980.

Pfeiffer R. Untersuchungen über das Choleragift. Zeitscher Hyg Infektionskr 11:393–412, 1892.

Pheils MT, Chapuis PH, Bokey EL, Hayward P. Diverticular disease: a retrospective study of surgical management 1970–1980. Aust NZ J Surg 52:53–56, 1982.

Pichlmayr R, Ziegler H. Die Relaparotomie bei Infektionen. Chirurg 45:208–216, 1974.

Pichlmayr R, Lehr, Pahlow J and Guthy E. Postoperative kontinuierliche dorso-ventrale Bauchspülung bei schweren Formen der Peritonitis. Chirurg 54:299–305, 1983.

Polk HC, Fry DE. Radical peritoneal debridement for established peritonitis. Ann Surg 192:350–355, 1980.

Pollack AV. Nonoperative antiinfective treatment of intraabdominal infections. World J Surg 14:227–230, 1990.

Pujol JP. La non fermature des incisions abdominales d'urgence. Techniques et résultats. Thèse de Médicine, Paris, U.E.R. X Bichat, 1975.

Bibliography

Pulverer G, Heinrich S, Infektionsversuche an Laboratoriumstierer und in vitro Untersuchungen zur Fermentausstattung des *Bacteroides melaninogenicus*. Zeitschr Hyg 146:341–349, 1960.

Raftery AT. Regeneration of perietal and visceral peritoneum: A light microscopical study. Br J Surg 60:293–299, 1973.

Raftery AT. Regeneration of perietal and visceral peritoneum: An electron microscopical study. J Anat 115:375–392, 1973.

Rangabashyam N: Peritonitis in India—Epidemiology, Mortality and Treatment Standards. In: DH Wittmann, JS Solomkin (eds): International Congress on Intraabdominal Infections, Hamburg, 1987.

Robinson SC. Observations on the peritoneum as an absorbing surface. Am J Obstet Gynecol 83:446–452, 1962.

Rotstein OD, Meakins JL. Diagnostic and therapeutic challenges of intraabdominal infections. World J Surg 14:159–166, 1990.

Rotstein OD, Pruet TL, Simmons RL. Microbiologic features and treatment of persistent peritonitis in patients in the intensive care unit. Can J Surg 29:247–250, 1986.

Runcie C, Ramsay G. Intraabdominal infection: pulmonary failure. World J Surg 14:196–203, 1990.

Sakai L, Daake J, Kaminski DL. Acute perforation of sigmoid diverticuli. Am J Surg 142:12–16, 1981.

Schein M, Saadia R, Decker GGA. The open management of the septic abdomen. Surg Gyn Obstet 163:587–592, 1986.

Schmidt H. Peritonitis. Behringwerk-Mitteilungen Heft 14. Schultz, Berlin, 1941, pp 58–79.

Schmitt HJ, Grinnan GLB. Use of Marlex mesh in infected abdominal war wound. Am J Surg 113:825–828, 1967.

Schoentag JJ, Platt ME, Cerra FB, Wels PB, Walzak P, Bukklay R. Aminoglycoside nephrotoxicity in critically ill surgical patients. J Surg Res 26:270–279, 1979.

Schreiber HW, Koch W, Diedrich K. Über die Bedeutung der Lymphographie beim Pfortaderhochdruck der Lebercirrhose. Langenbecks Arch Klin Chir 317:124–129, 1967.

Schreiber HW, von Ackeren H, Rehnmer M, Schilling K. Sep-

tische Erkrankungen der Bauchhöhle. Chirurg 42:346–352, 1971.

Schwaiger N. Postoperative peritonitis. Langenbecks Arch Klin Chir 247:411–414, 1978.

Simmons RL. Intra-abdominal abscesses: principles governing treatment. The Upjohn Company, 1981.

Simmons RL, Howard RL. Surgical infectious diseases. Appleton-Century-Crofts, New York, 1982.

Simmons RL, Ahrenholz, DH. Pathobiology of peritonitis: a review. J Antimicrob Chemother 7:A29–36, 1981.

Solomkin JS, Simmons RL: Candida infection in surgical patients. World J Surg 4:381, 1980.

Solomkin JS, Bauman MP, Nelson RD, Simmons RL. Neutrophil dysfunction during the course of intraabdominal infection. Ann Surg 194:9–17, 1981.

Solomkin JS, Meakins JL, All MD, et al.: Antibiotics trials in intra-abdominal infections: a critical evaluation of study design and outcome reporting. Ann Surg 200:29–39, 1984.

Spitzy KH. Zur Behandlung chronischer chirurgischer Infektionen. Chirurg 38:165–168, 1967.

Stahl TJ, Cerra FB: Hemodynamic and metabolic responses to infection. In: RL Simmons, RJ Howar (eds): Surgical Infectious Disease. 2nd ed. Appleton-Century-Crofts, New York, 1989 pp 209–232.

Steinberg D. On leaving the peritoneal cavity open in acute generalized suppurative peritonitis. Am J Surg 137:216–220, 1979.

Stephen M, Loewenthal K. Generalized infective peritonitis. Surg Gynecol Obstet 147:231–235, 1978.

Stille W. Chemotherapeutic aspects of anaerobic septicemia. Infection 8:S191–192, 1979.

Stone HH, Kolb LD, Geheber CE. Incidence and significance of intraperitoneal anaerobic bacteria. Ann Surg 181:705–715, 1975.

Stone HH, Storm PR, Mullins RJ. Pancreatic abscess management by subtotal resection and packing. World J Surg 8:340–345, 1984.

Strauss AA. A new method and end results in the treatment of carcinoma of the stomach and rectum by surgical diathermy. JAMA 106:285–286, 1936.

Stremmel W. Drainagebehandlung

ohne Antibiotica. Langenbecks Arch Chir 347:415, 1979.

Sudek (zit, nach Wachsmuth, 1965).

Swenson RM, Lorber B, Michaelson TC, Spaulding EH. The bacteriology of intra-abdominal infections. Arch Surg 109:398–399, 1974.

Taenaeus A, Heimbürger O, Lindholm B. Peritonitis during continuous peritoneal lavage (CAPD): risk factors, clinical severity, and pathogenic aspects. Peritoneal Dial Int 8:253, 1987.

Teichmann W, Eggert A, Kirschner H, Herden N. Die Etappenlavage bei diffuser Peritonitis. Chirurg 53:374–376, 1982.

Teichmann W, Eggert A, Wittmann DH, Böcker W. Der Reissverschluss als neue Methode des temporären Bauchdeckenverschlusses in der Abdominalchirurgie. Chirurg 56:173–178, 1985.

Teichmann W, Wittmann DH, Andreone A. Scheduled reoperations (Etappenlavage) for diffuse peritonitis. Arch Surg 121:147–152, 1986.

Trede M, Lampe H-J, Linder M, Wesch G. Peritonitis in hohen Lebensalter. In: R Häring (ed): Peritonitis. TM-Verlag, Bad Oeynhausen, 1979, pp 173–179.

Trede M, Linder MM, Wesch G. Die Indikation zur relaparotomie bei postopserativer peritonitis. Langenbecks Arch Klin Chir 352:295, 1980.

Trede M, Linder MM, Wesh G. Die Indikation zur Relaparotomie bei postoperativer Peritonitis. Langenbecks Arch Chir 352:295–299, 1983.

Tsilibary EC, Wissig SL. Absorption from the peritoneal cavity: SEM study of the mesothelium covering the peritoneal surface of the muscular portion of the diaphragm. Am J Anat 149:127–133, 1977.

VanDijk WC. *Escherichia coli* infections. Microbial virulence factors and phagocytic cell defense. Habilitationsschrift der Rijksuniversiteit te Utrecht, 1980.

von Recklinghausen FT. Die Lymphgefäβe und ihre Bindegewebe. Hirschwald, Berlin, 1862.

Wachsmuth W. Peritonitis. Langenbecks Arch Klin Chir 313:146–169, 1965.

Wang MS, Wilson SE. Subphrenic abscess. The new epidemiology. Arch Surg 112:934–936, 1976.

Wegner G. Chirurgische Bemerkungen über die Peritonealhöhle mit besonderer Berücksichtigung der Ovariotomie. Arch Klin Chir 20:51–145, 1876.

Weinstein WM, Onderdonk AB, Bartlett JG, Gorbach SL. Experimental intra-abdominal abscesses in rats: development of an experimental model. Infect Immunol 10:1250–1255, 1974.

Weissenhofer W. Antisepsis in der Behandlung der diffusen bakteriellen Bauchfellentzündung. Acta Chir Austriaca Suppl 31:3–20, 1979.

Welter J, Wittmann DH. Peritonitis der alten Menschen. In: P Kempf (ed): Behandlung der Peritonitis. Zuckschwerdt, Munich, 1980, pp 155–165.

Werner B. Thoracic duct cannulation in man: I. Surgical technique and a clinical study on 79 patients. Acta Chir Scand 353(Suppl):S1–24, 1965.

Werner H. Mikrobiologische Aspekte der Peritonitis. In: P Kempf (ed): Behandlung der Peritonitis. Zuckschwerdt, Munich, 1980, pp 49–53.

Werner H. Anaerobierinfektionen. Thieme, Stuttgart, 1981.

Wilson SE. Secondary bacterial peritonitis. In: SE Wilson, SM Finegold, RA Williams (eds): Intra-abdominal Infection. McGraw-Hill, New York, 1982, pp 62–88.

Wilson SE. Intra-abdominal abscess. In: SE Wilson, SM Finegold, RA Williams (eds): Intra-abdominal infection. McGraw-Hill, New York, 1982, pp 172–206.

Wittmann DH, Welter J, Schassan H-H. Untersuchung über die Penetration von β-Lactam-Antibiotika in das Peritonealexsudat als Grundlage der systemischen Peritonitistherapie. In: R Häring (ed): Peritonitis. TM-Verlag, Bad Oeynhausen, 1979, pp 85–92.

Wittmann DH. Beteiligung von anaeroben Keimen bei Gallenwegsin-fektionen. In: R Häring (ed): Peritonitis. TM-Verlag, Bad Oeynhausen, 1979, pp 83–84.

Wittmann DH. Chemotherapeutic principles of difficult-to-treat infections in surgery: I. Peritonitis. Infection 8:323–329, 1980.

Wittmann DH, Schassan H-H, Freitag V. Über die Korrelation pharmakokinetisch-bakteriologischer Befunde mit den klinischen Resultaten der antimikrobiellen Chemotherapie der Peritonitis. In: B Wiedemann (ed): Die Resistenz gegenüber β-lactam-Antibiotika. Paul-Ehrlich-Gesellschaft, Bad Honnef, 1980, pp 242–249.

Wittmann DH. Pharmakokinetische Grundlagen chirurgischer Infektionen. Zbl Chir 106:1231, 1981.

Wittmann DH, Teichmann W, Adam D, Rubinstein E, Eggert A. A new method of measuring the protein unbound fraction of antibiotics in the peritoneal cavity. Program and Abstract of the 21st Interscience Conference on Antimicrobial Agents and Chemotherapy, American Society for Microbiology, Abstr 102, 1981.

Wittmann DH. Chemotherapeutische Grundsätze bei Infektionsproblemen in der Chirurgie: Intraabdominelle Infektionen. Acta Chir Austriaca Suppl 43:22–23, 1982.

Wittmann DH. Grundlagen der antimikrobiellen Peritonitistherapie. Langenbecks Arch Chir 358:589, 1982.

Wittmann DH, Welter J. Oberbauchperitonitis. In: P Kempf (ed): Behandlung der Peritonitis. Zuckschwerdt, Munich, 1982, pp 155–165.

Wittmann DH (Ed). Intraabdominelle Infektionen. Fortschr Antimikrob Antineoplast Chemother (FAC) Bd. 2–3. Futuramed, Munich, 1983.

Wittmann DH. Grundlagen zur kalkulierten Chemotherapie intraabdomineller Infektionen. In: DH Wittmann (ed): Intraabdominelle Infektionen. Fortschr Antimikrob Antineoplast Chemother (FAC) Bd. 2–3. Futuramed, Munich, 1983, pp 467–478.

Wittmann DH, Kellinghusen C, Frommelt L. Peritonitis nach Sigmadivertikelperforation. In: DH Wittmann (ed): Intraabdominelle Infektionen. Fortschr Antimikrob Antineoplast Chemother (FAC) Bd. 2–3. Furturamed, Munich, 1983, pp 535–542.

Wittmann DH, Frommelt L. Metronidazol bei intraabdominellen Infektionen. In: DH Wittmann (ed): Intraabdominelle Infektionen. Fortschr Antimikrob Antineoplast Chemother (FAC) Bd. 2–3. Furturamed, Munich, 1983, pp 703–706.

Wittmann DH, Kellinghusen C, Welter J, Freitag V. Intraabdominelle Infektionen: Ergebnisse einer kontrollierten Therapiestudie. Akt Chir 18:229–353, 1983.

Wittmann DH, Schassan HH. Penetration of eight β-lactam antibiotics into the peritoneal fluid. Arch Surg 118:205–212, 1983.

Wittmann DH. Zur Therapie der Bauchfellentzündung: Die Komentrationsdynamik am Infektionsort also Bewertungskriterium der antimikrobiellen Chemotherapie. Habilitationsschrift der Universität Hamburg, 1984.

Wittmann DH, Teichmann W, Frommelt L. The impact of intra-abdominal pathogens on treatment of purulent peritonitis. (In German). Chirurg 56:363–370, 1985.

Wittmann DH and Teichmann W. Therapy for pathogenic bacteria in diffuse peritonitis by scheduled relaparotomies. Langenbecks Arch Chir 366:629, 1985.

Wittmann DH, Müller, M. The PIAII Score for intra-abdominal infections. In Workbook of International Congress on Intra-abdominal Infections. Adelphi Communications, Macclesfield, Cheshire, pp 19–21, 1987.

Wittmann DH, Teichmann W, Müller M. Development and validation of the Peritonitis-Index-Altona (PIA II). Langenbecks Arch Chir 372:834–835, 1987.

Wittmann DH, Aprahamian C, Bergstein JM. A temporary device for abdominal closure. Surg Gyn Obstet. In preparation, 1990.

Wittmann DH. Etappenlavage: Advanced diffuse peritonitis managed by planned multiple laparotomies utilizing zippers, slide fastener, and Velcro for temporary abdominal closure. World J Surg 14:218–226, 1990.

Wittmann DH. Intraabdominal infections—Introduction. World J Surg 14:145–147, 1990.

Wittmann DH, Nystrom PO. Multicentre validation of Apache II Score in intra-abdominal infection. Surg Res Commun 8:27, 1990.

Wouters DB, Krom RAF, Slooff MJH, Kootstra G, Kuijjer PJ. The use of Marlex mesh in patients with generalized peritonitis and multiple organ system failure. Surg Gyn Obstet 156:609–614, 1983.

Index